MW01382334

Printed in the United States of America

Published by ACB | Adult Coloring Books

ISBN 978-1-988245-22-5

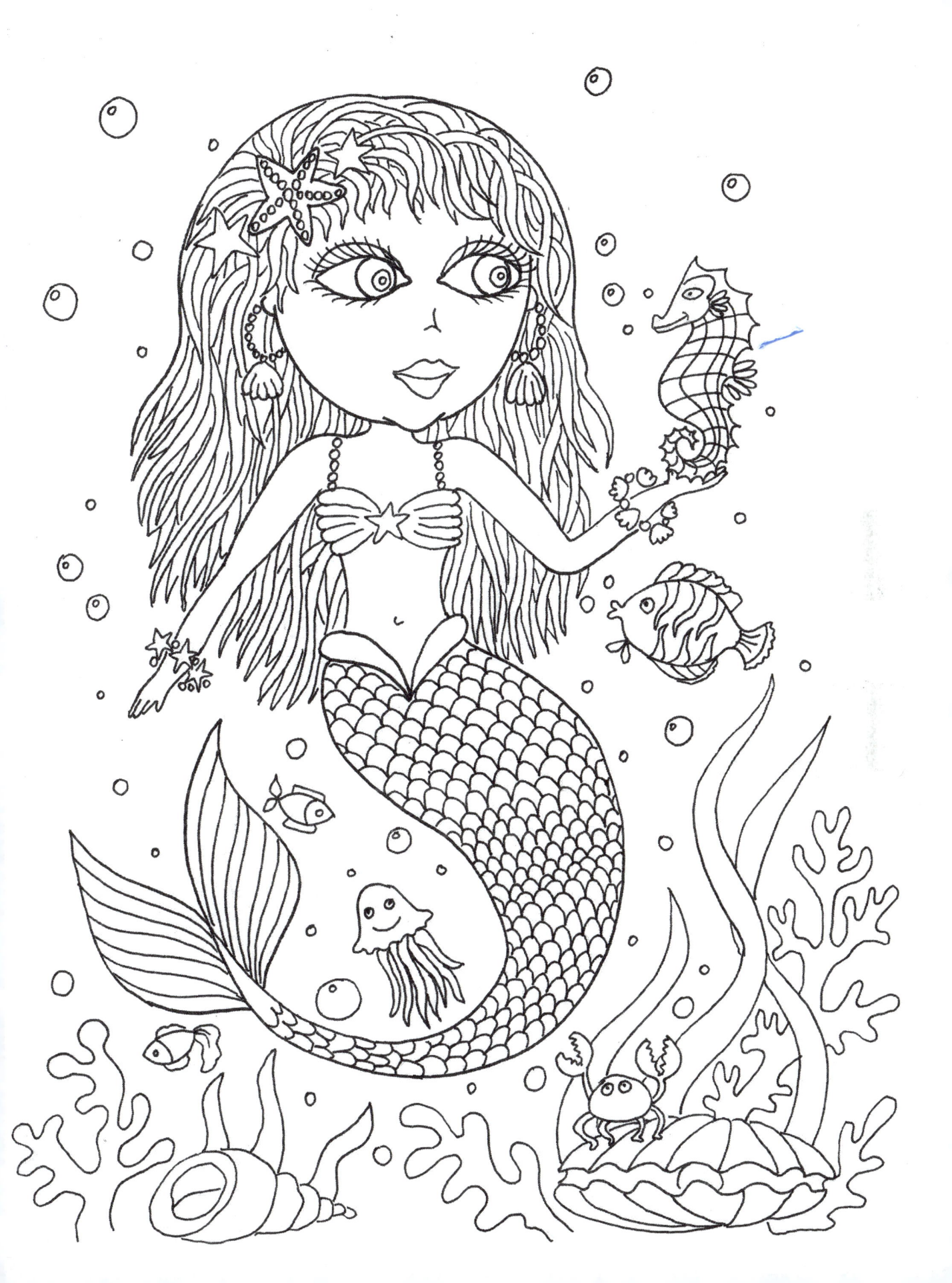

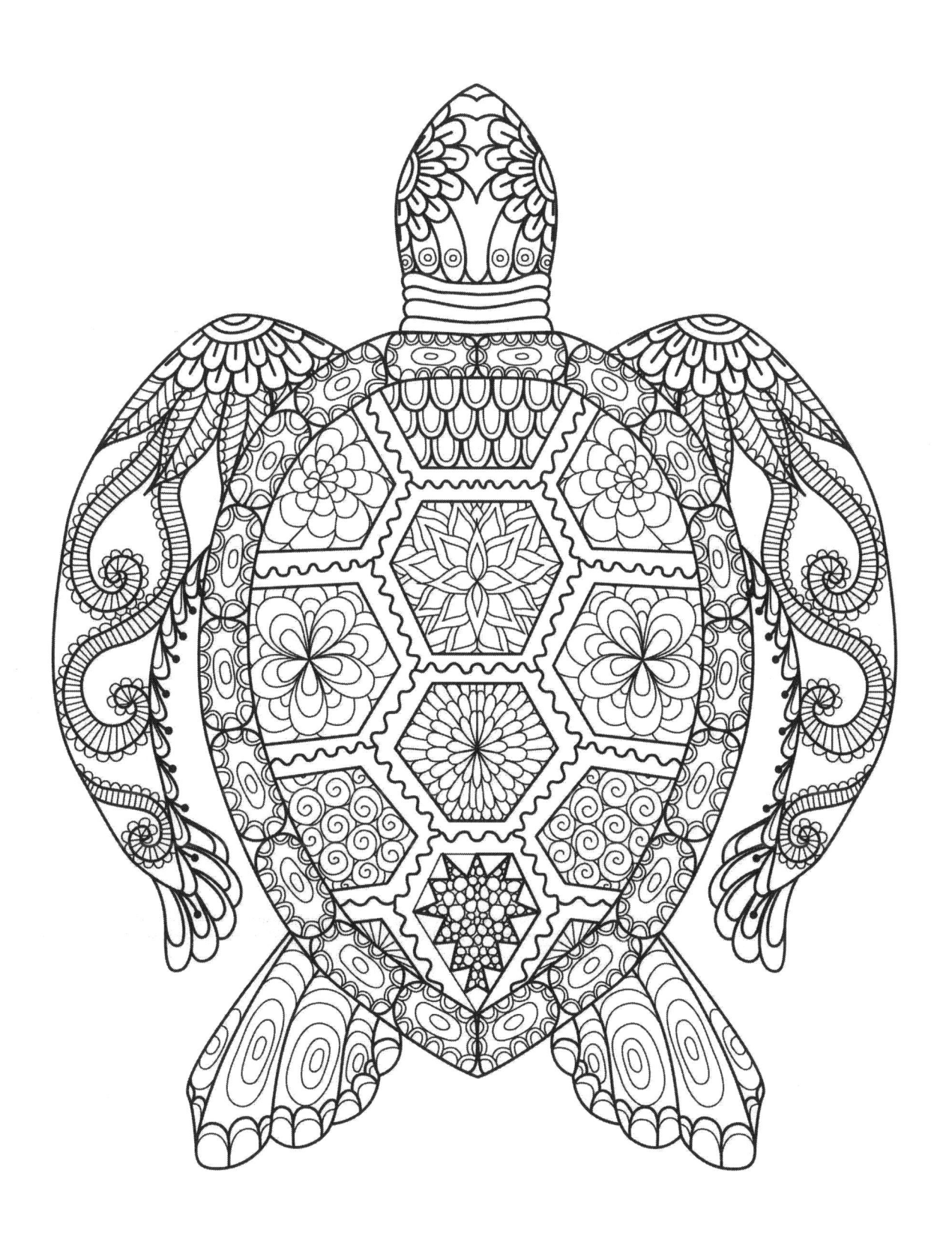

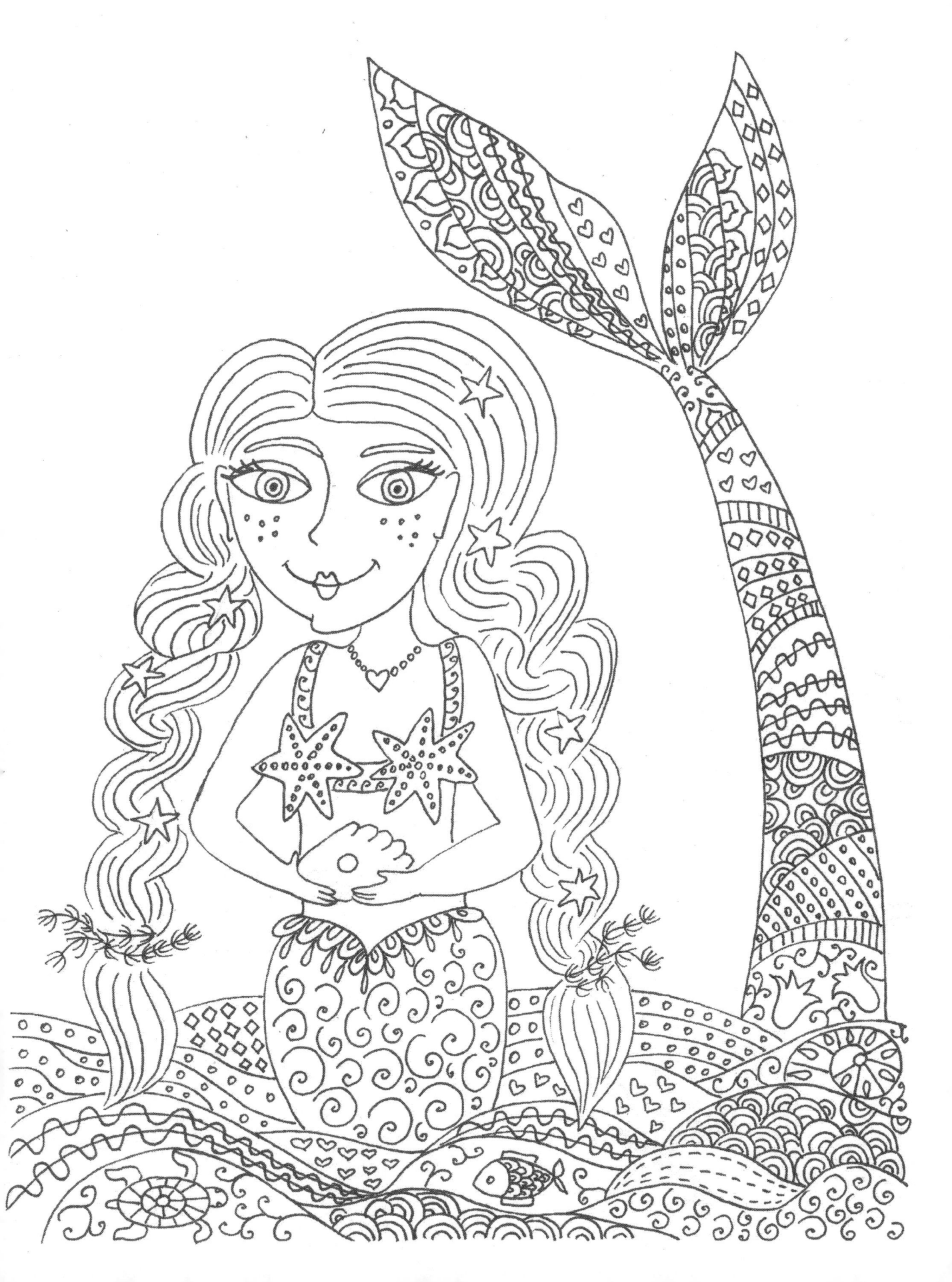

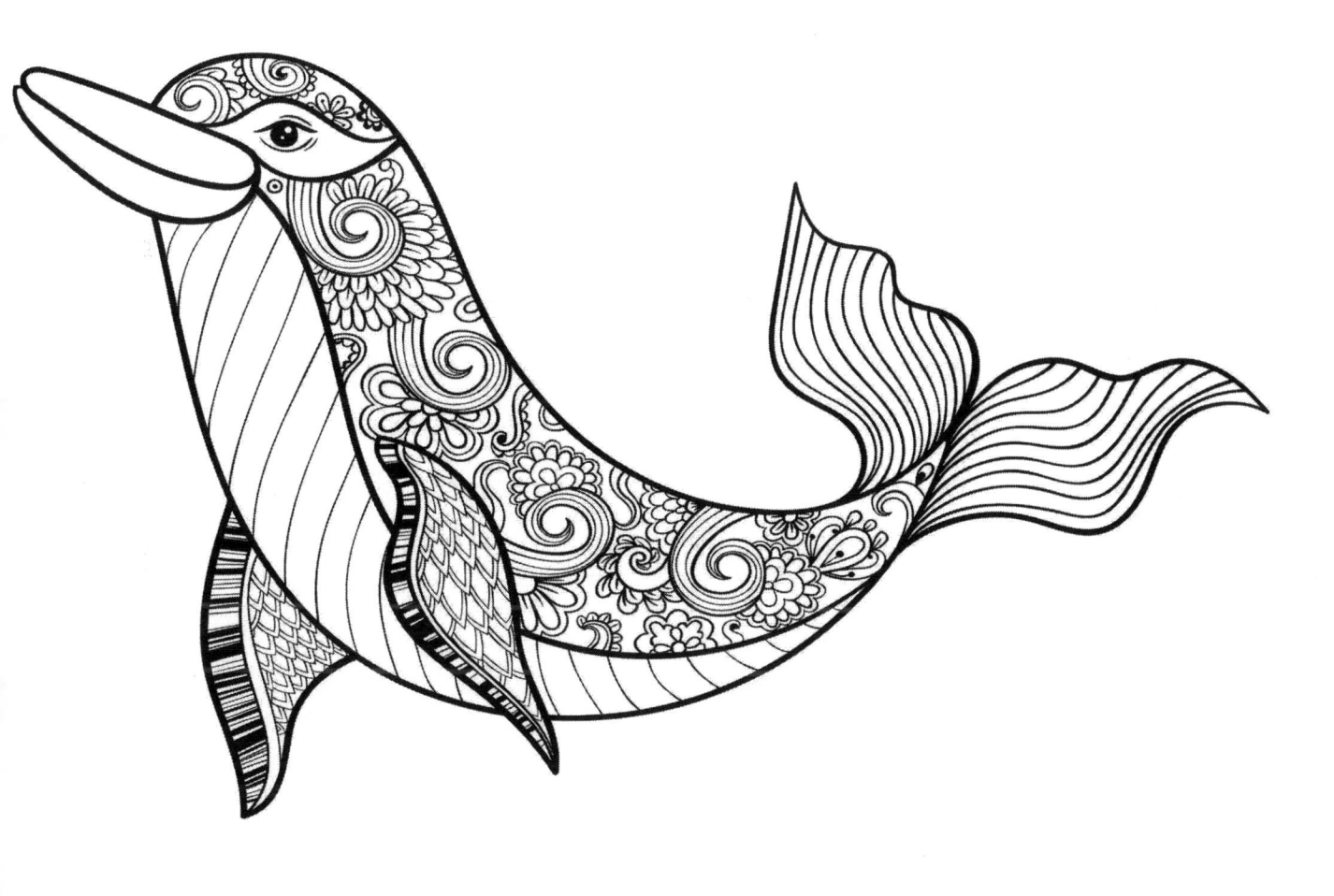

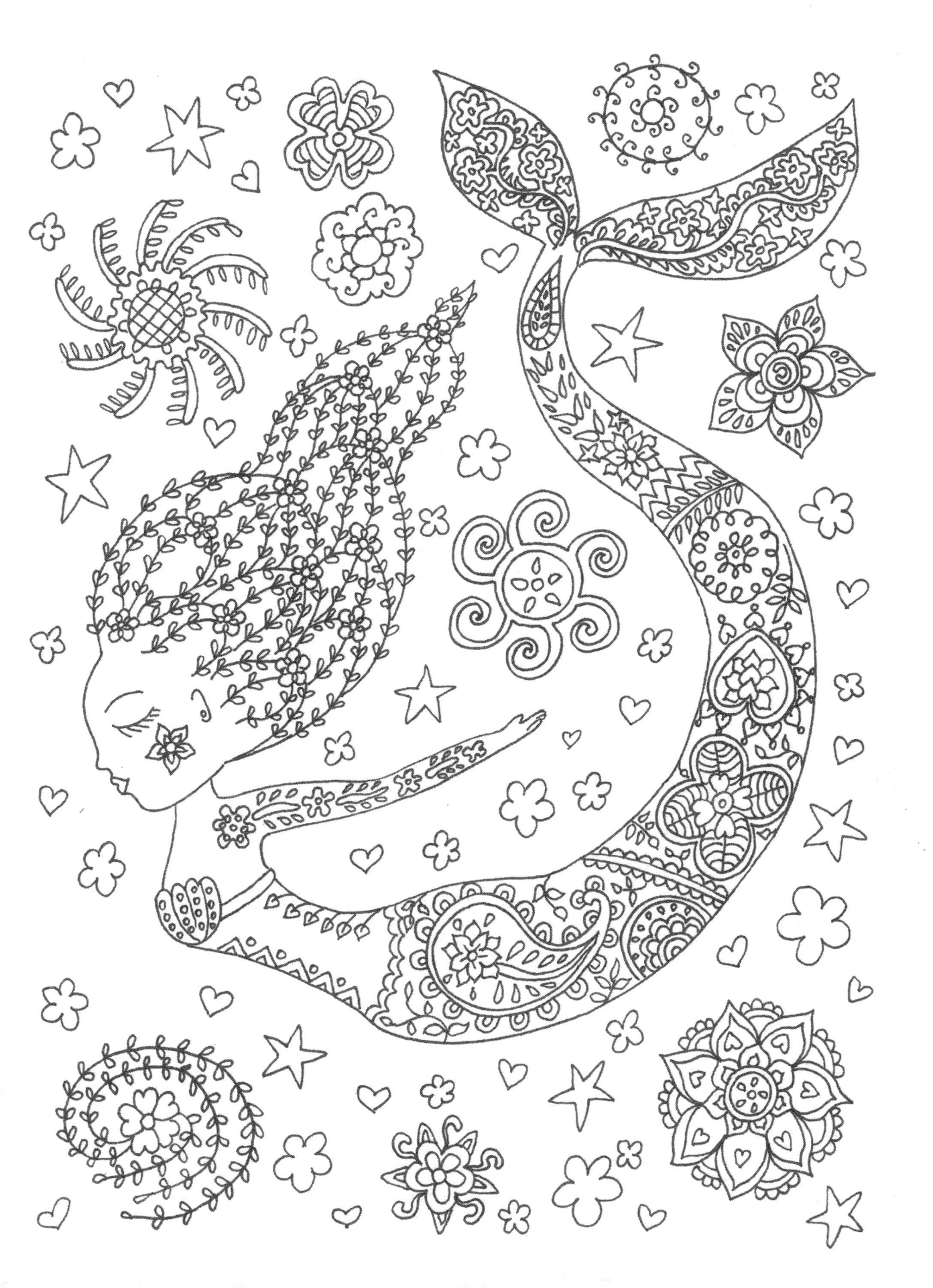

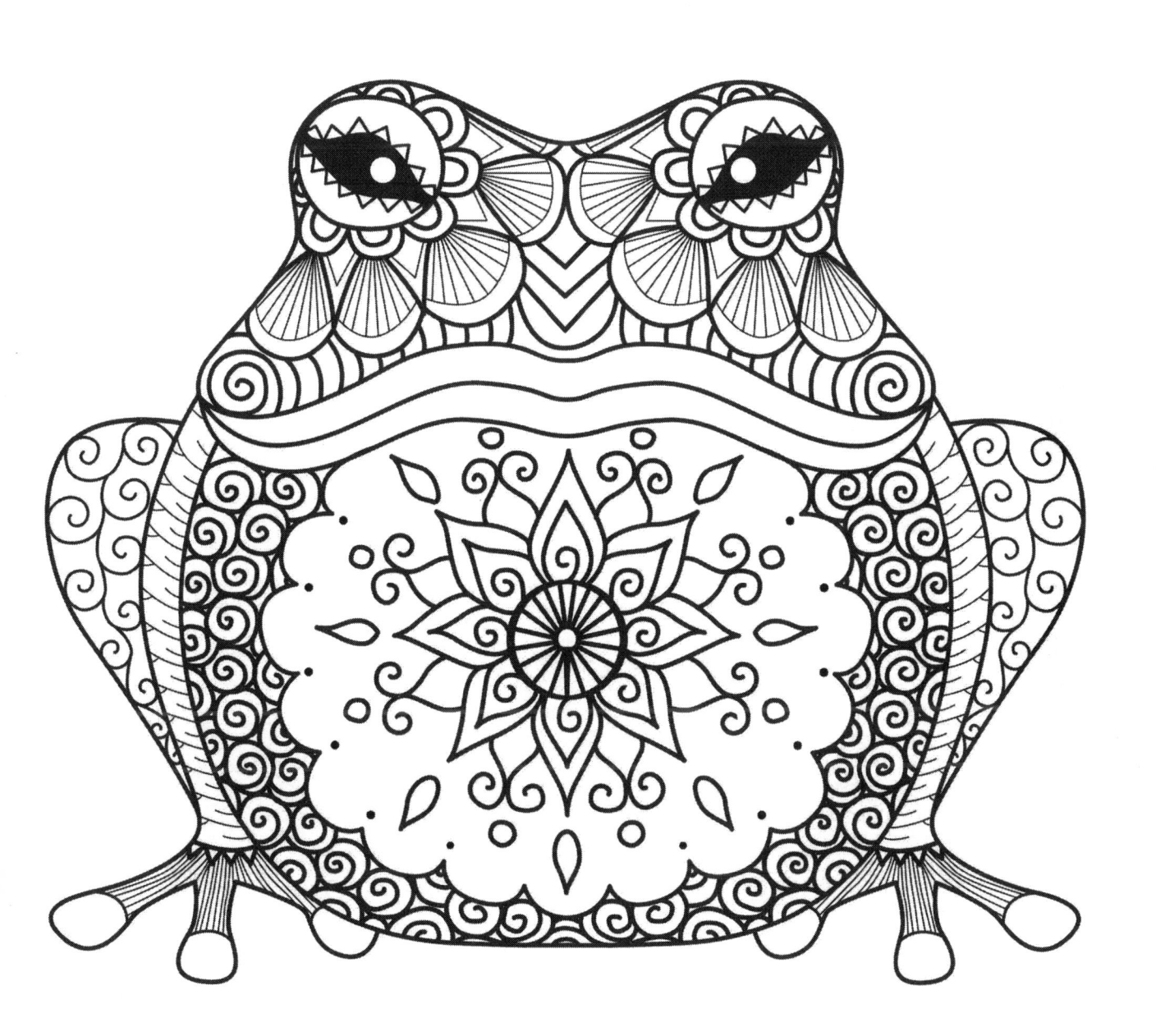

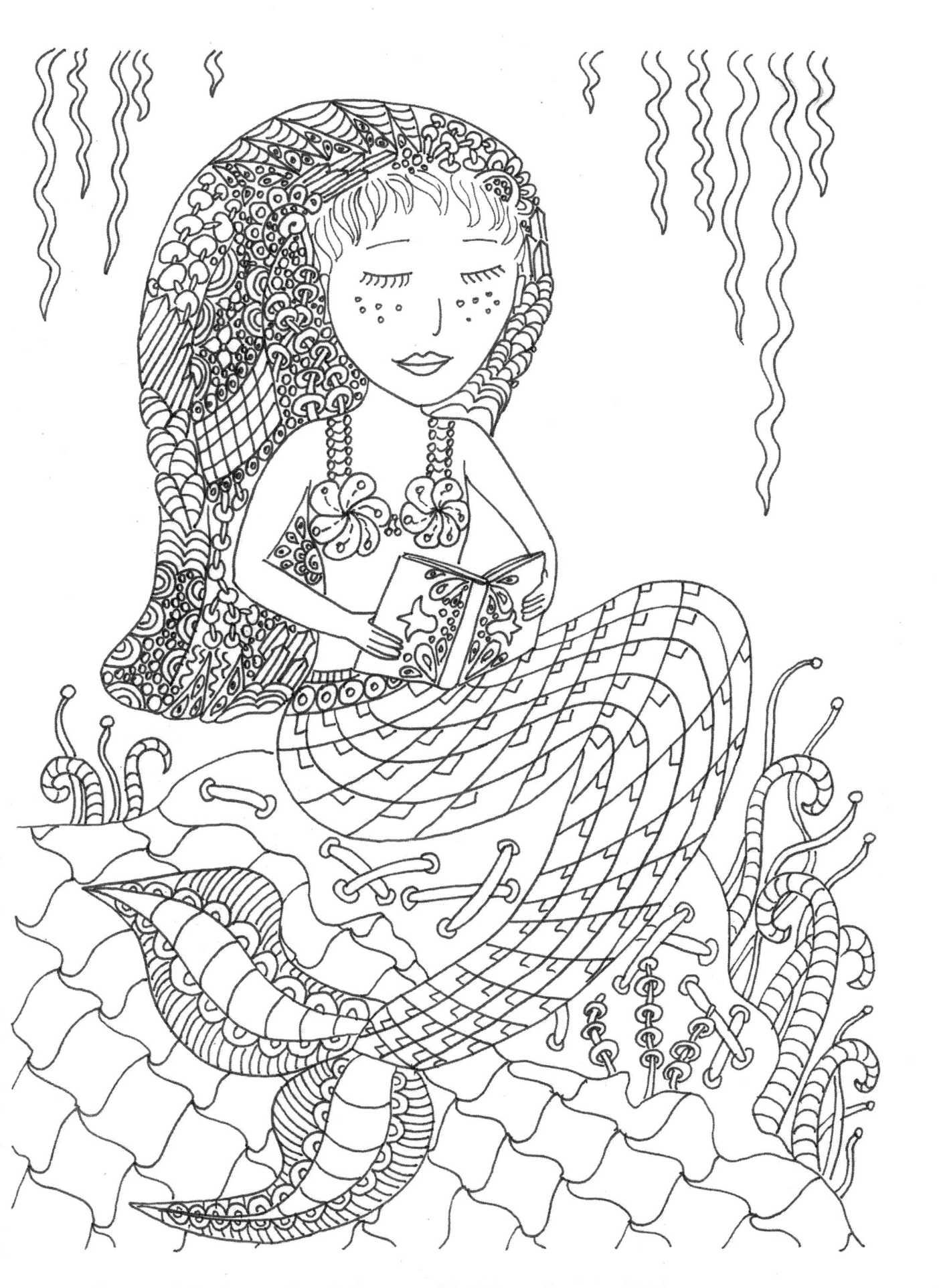

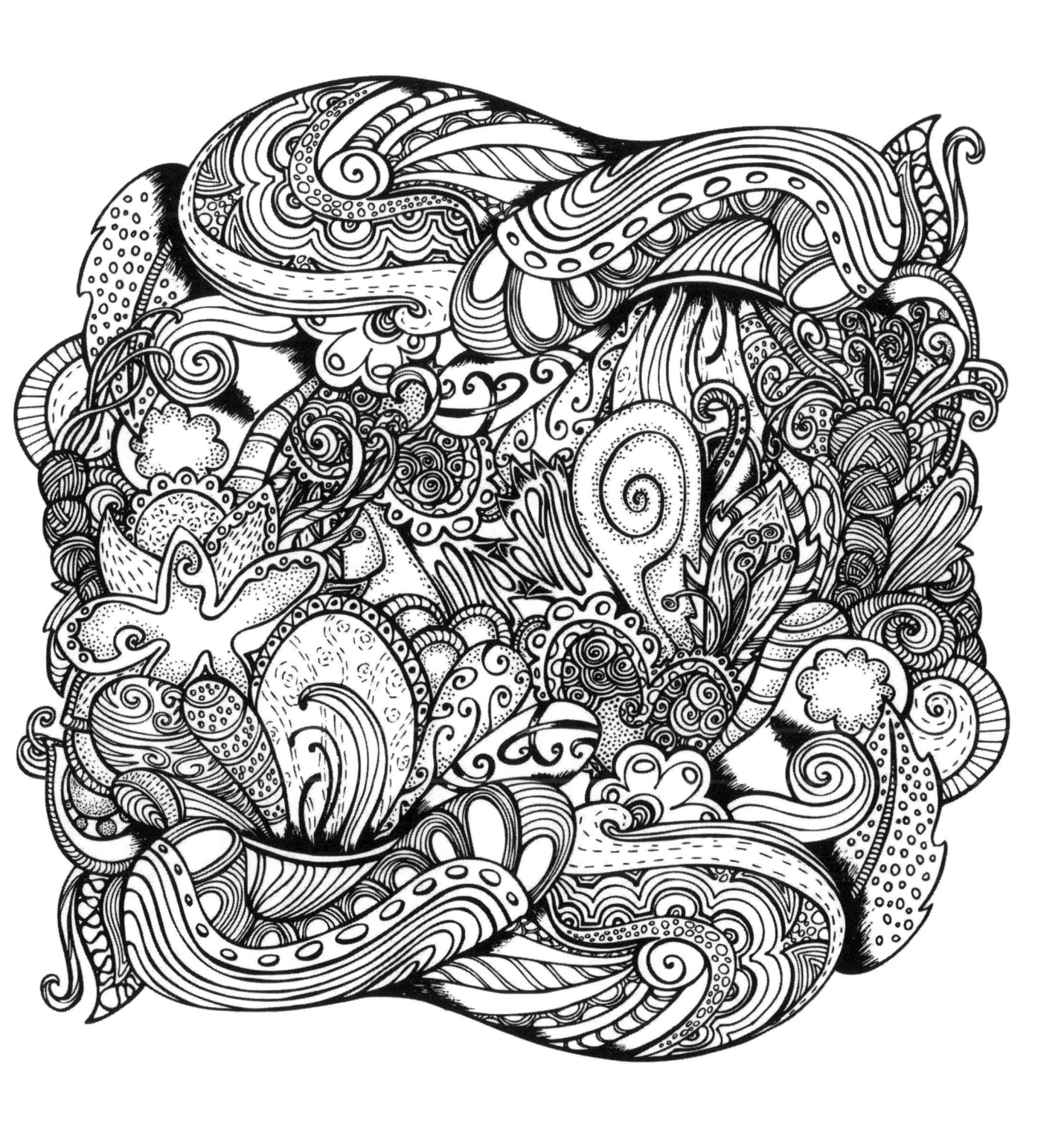

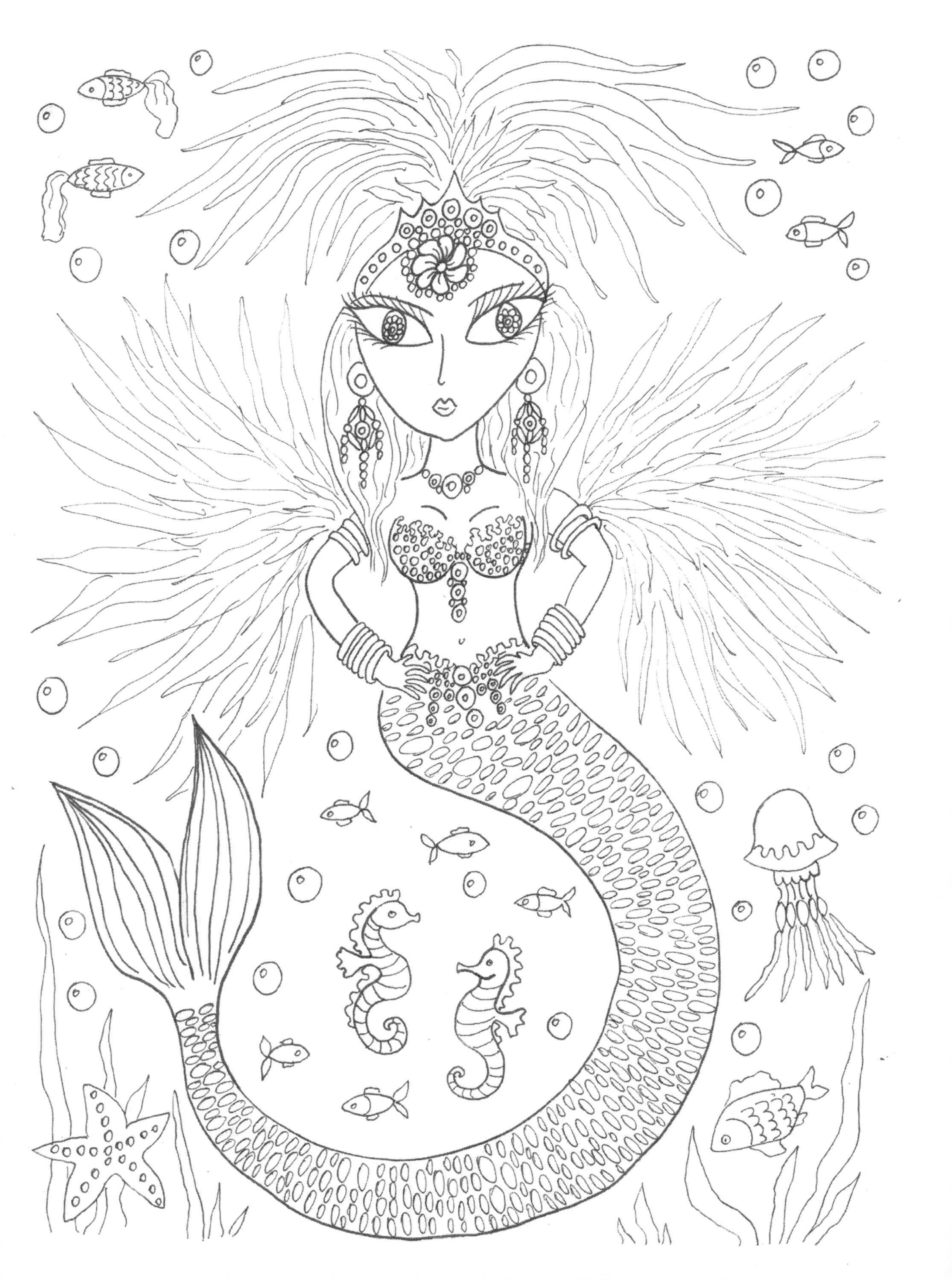

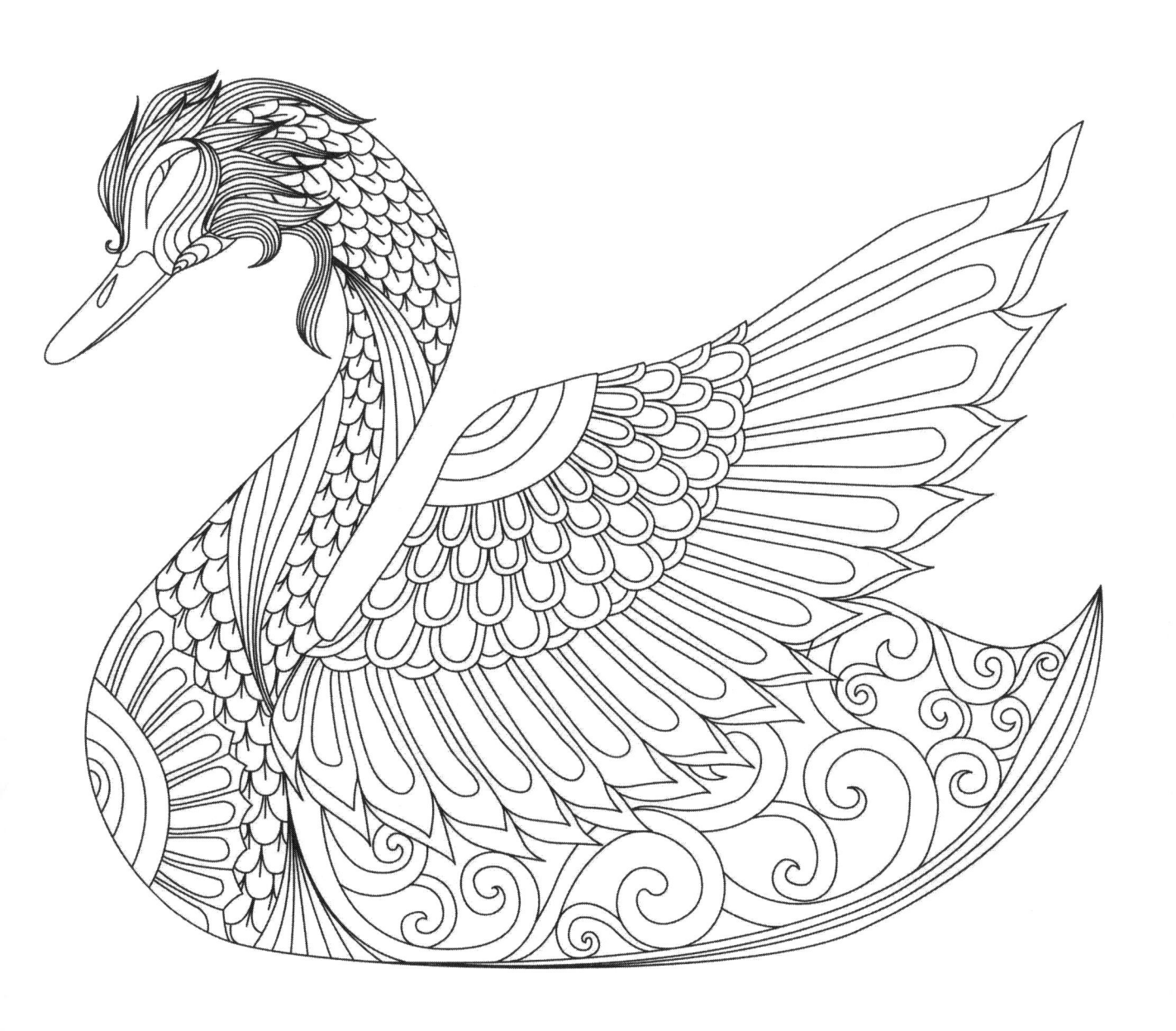

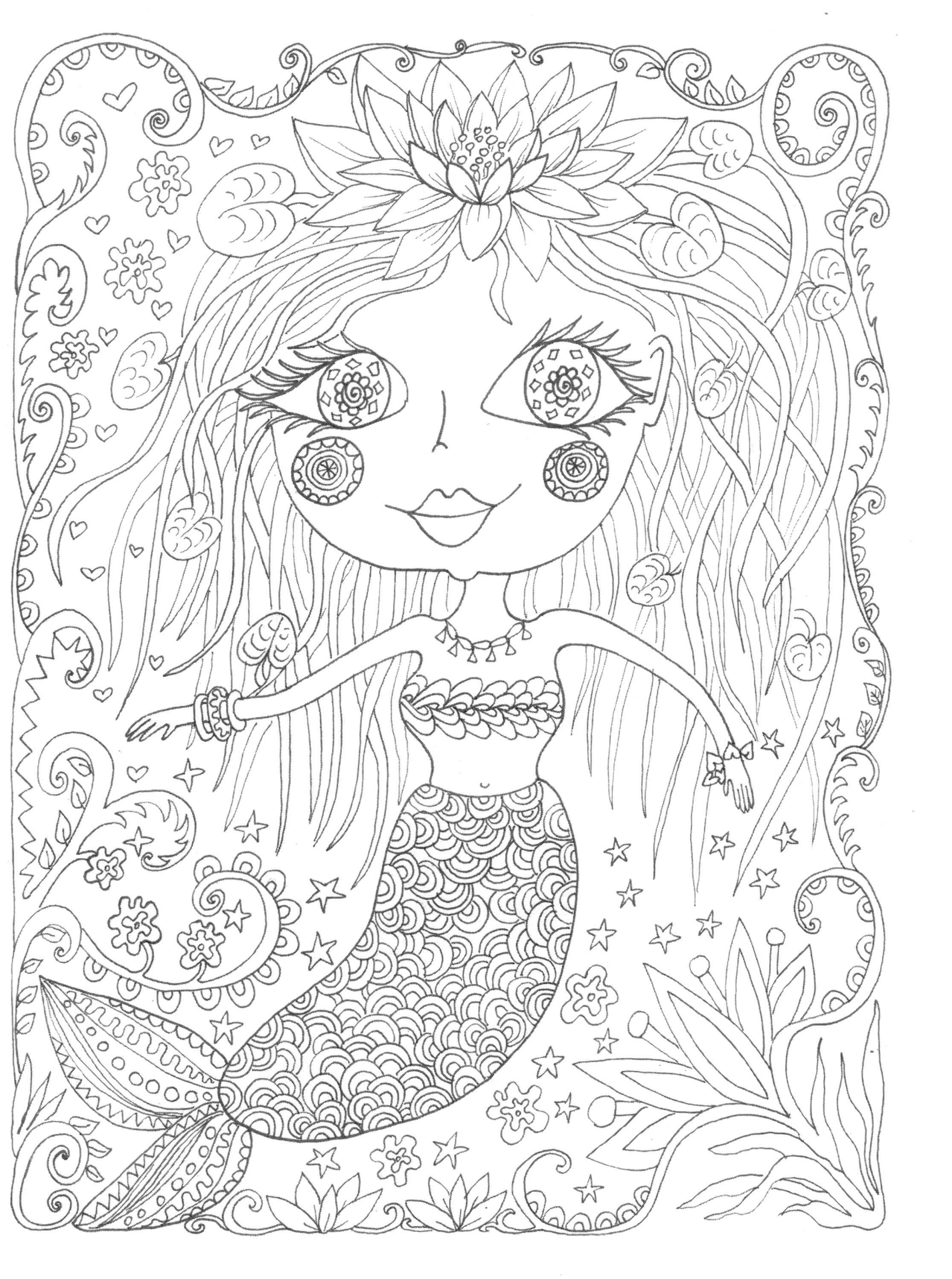

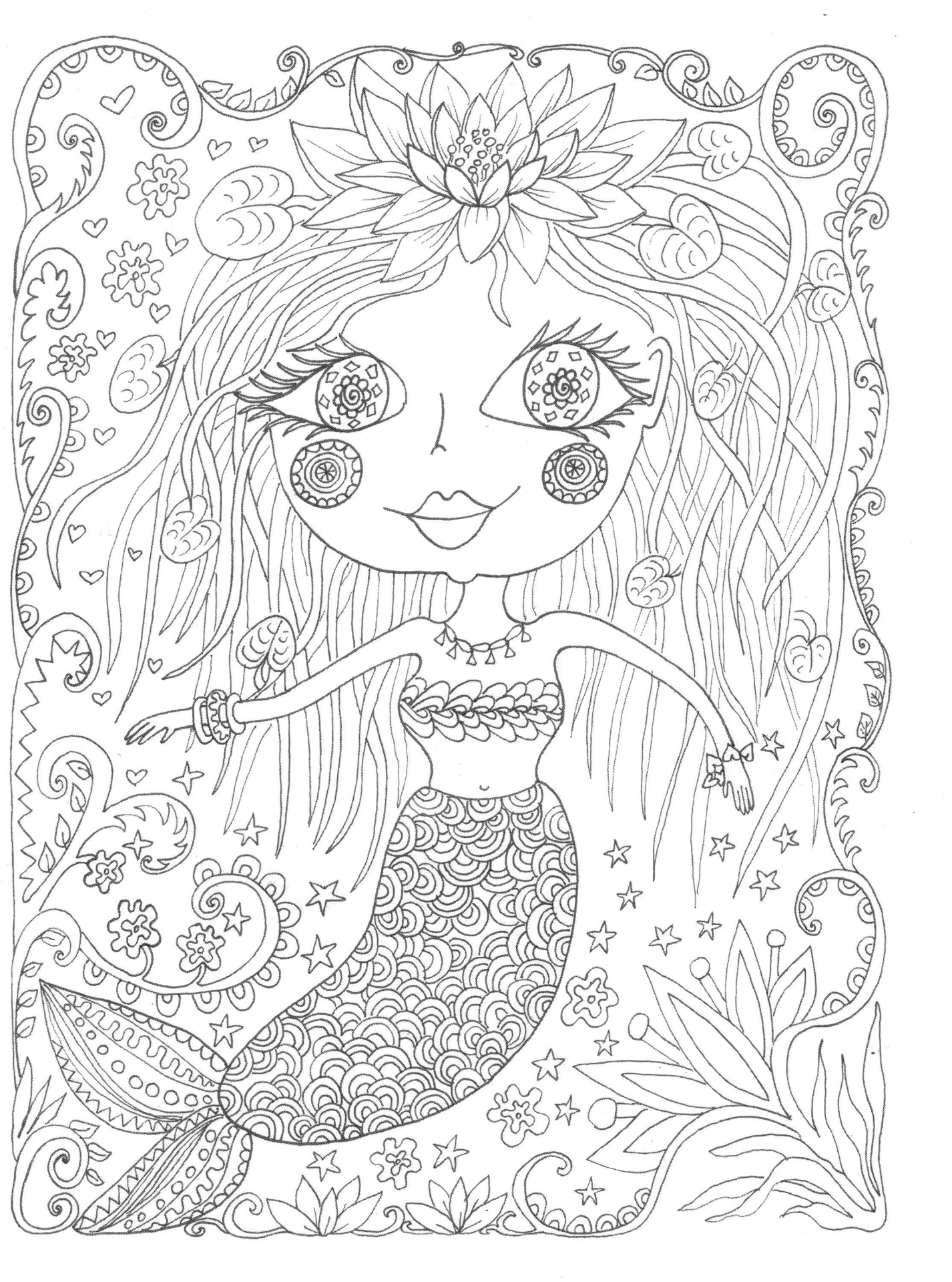

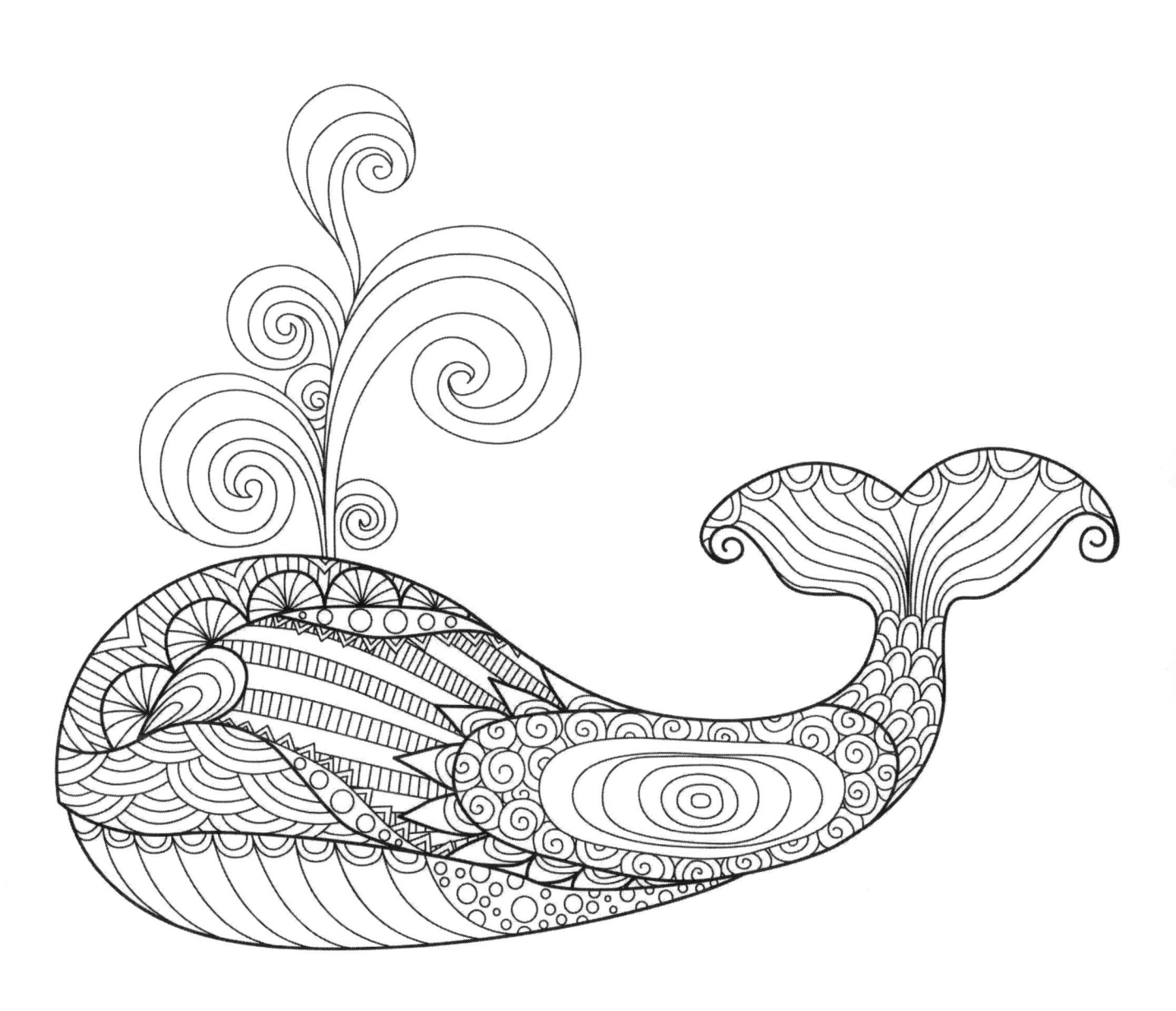

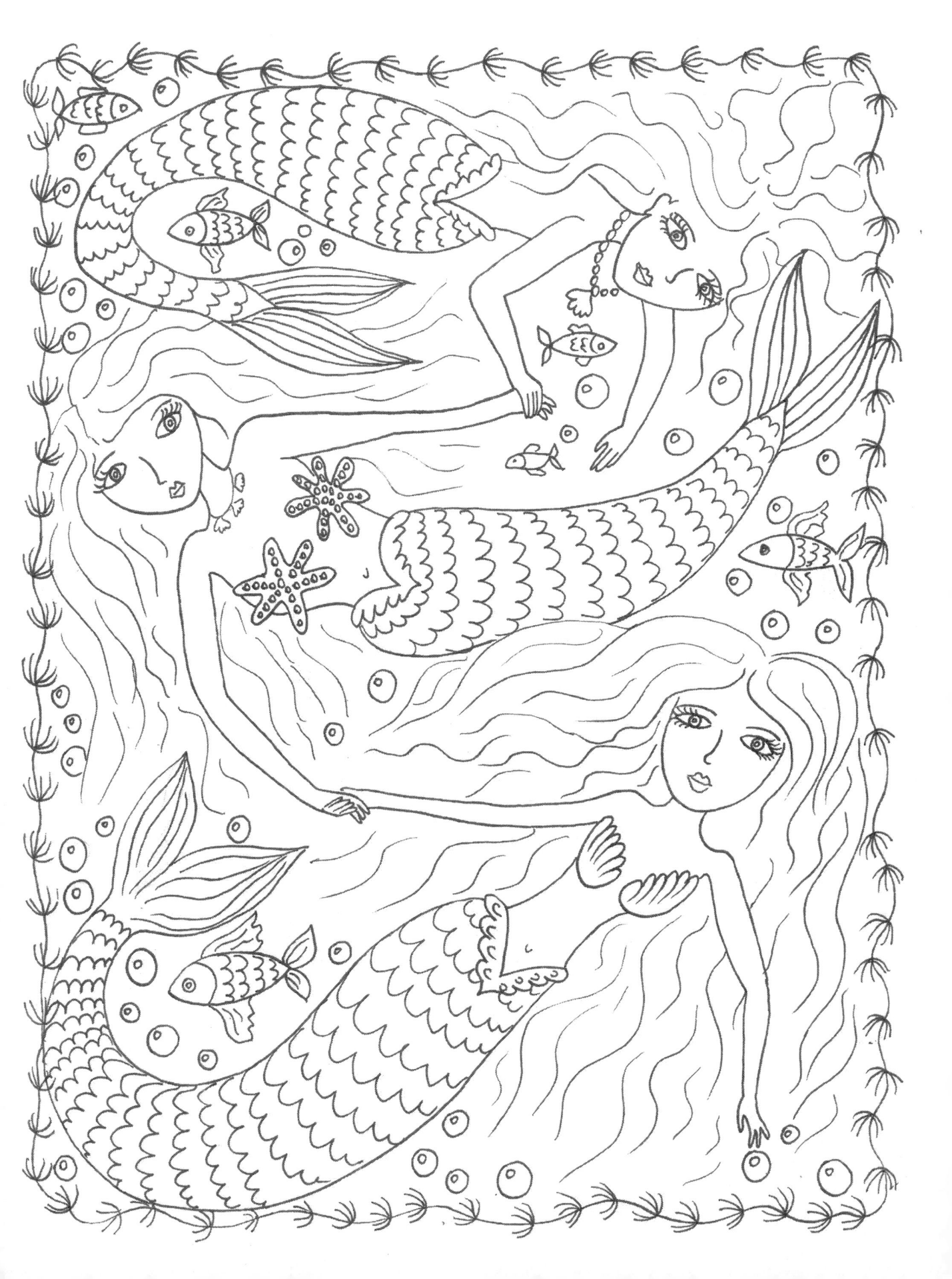

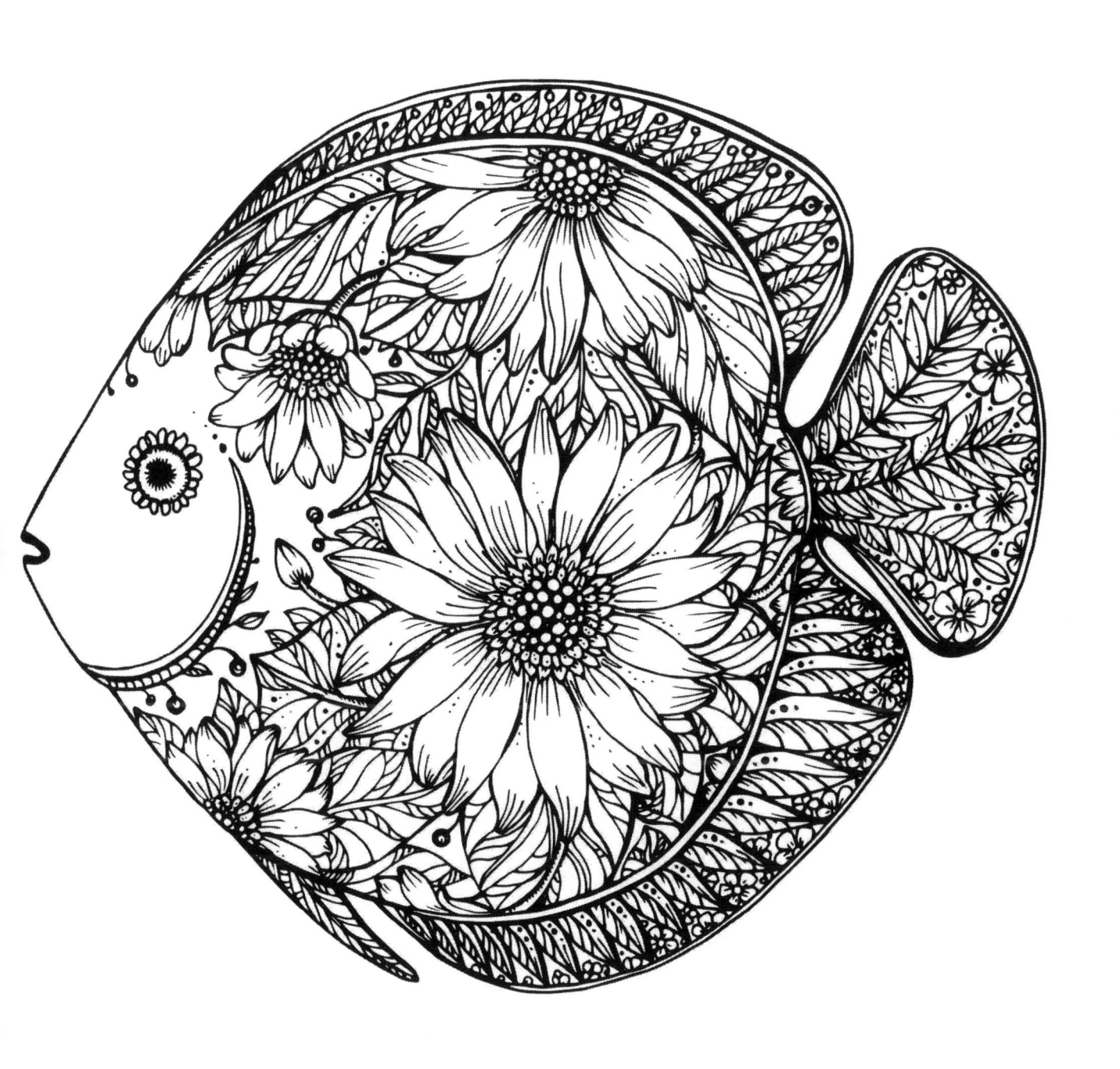

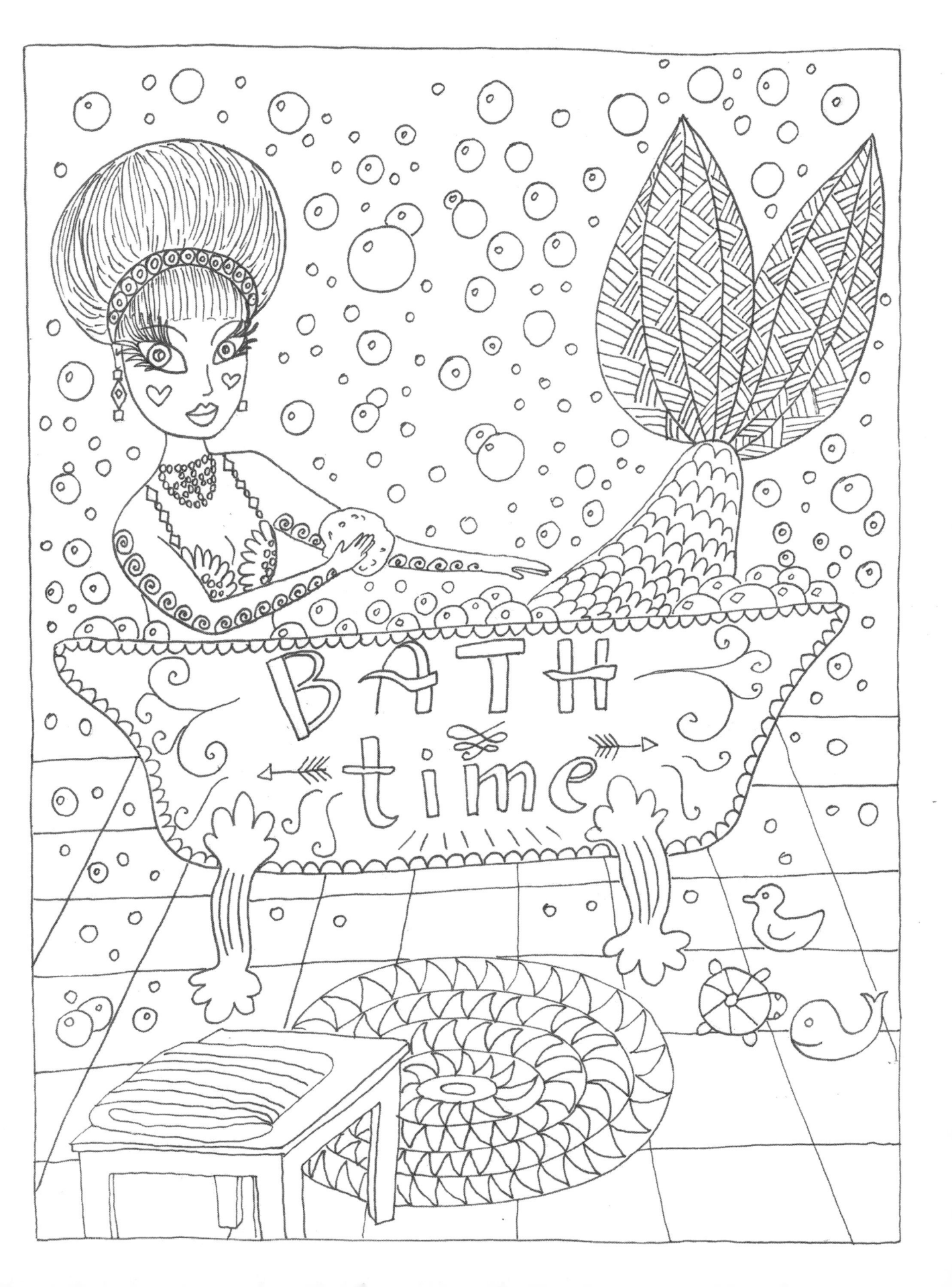

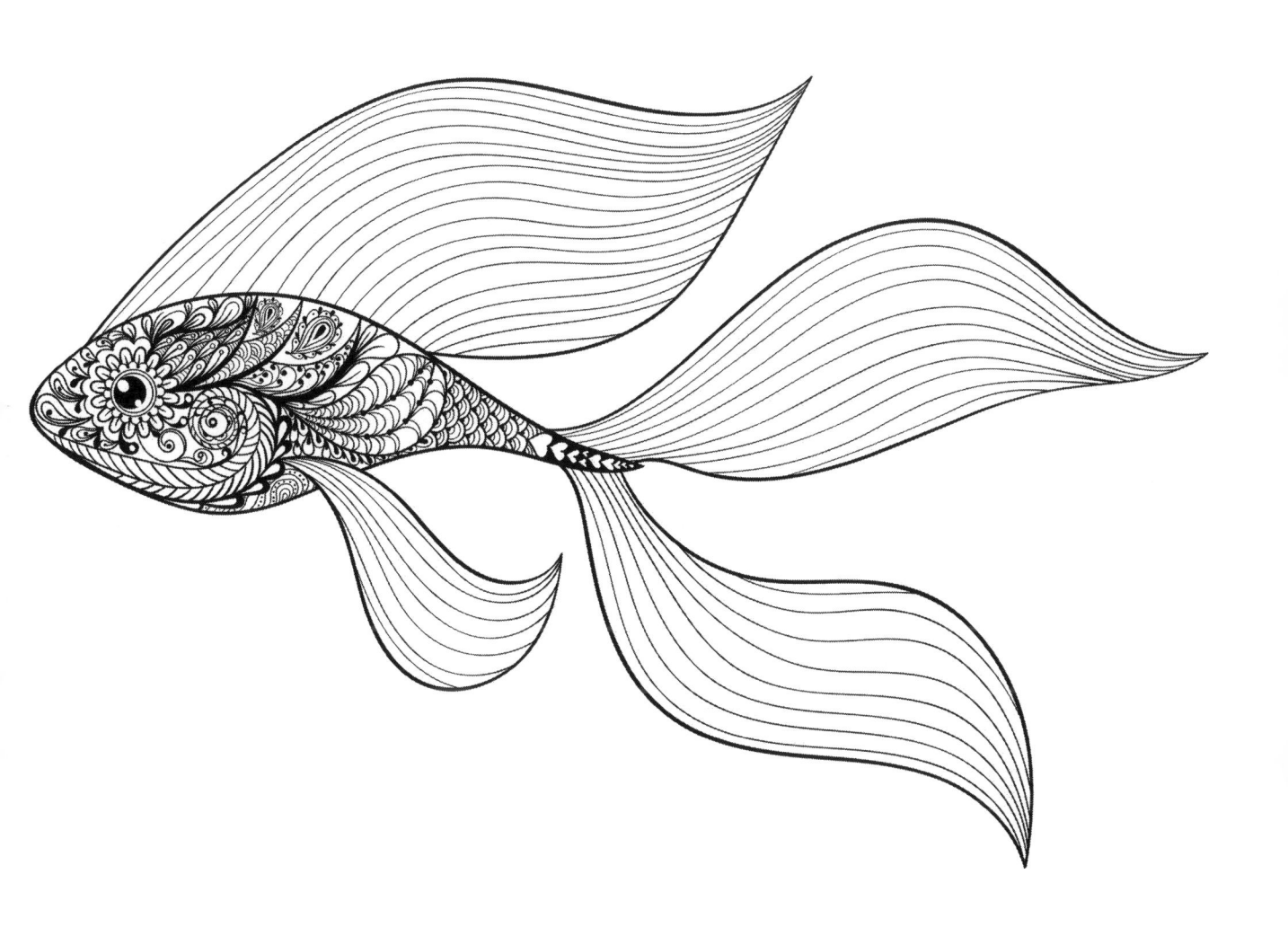

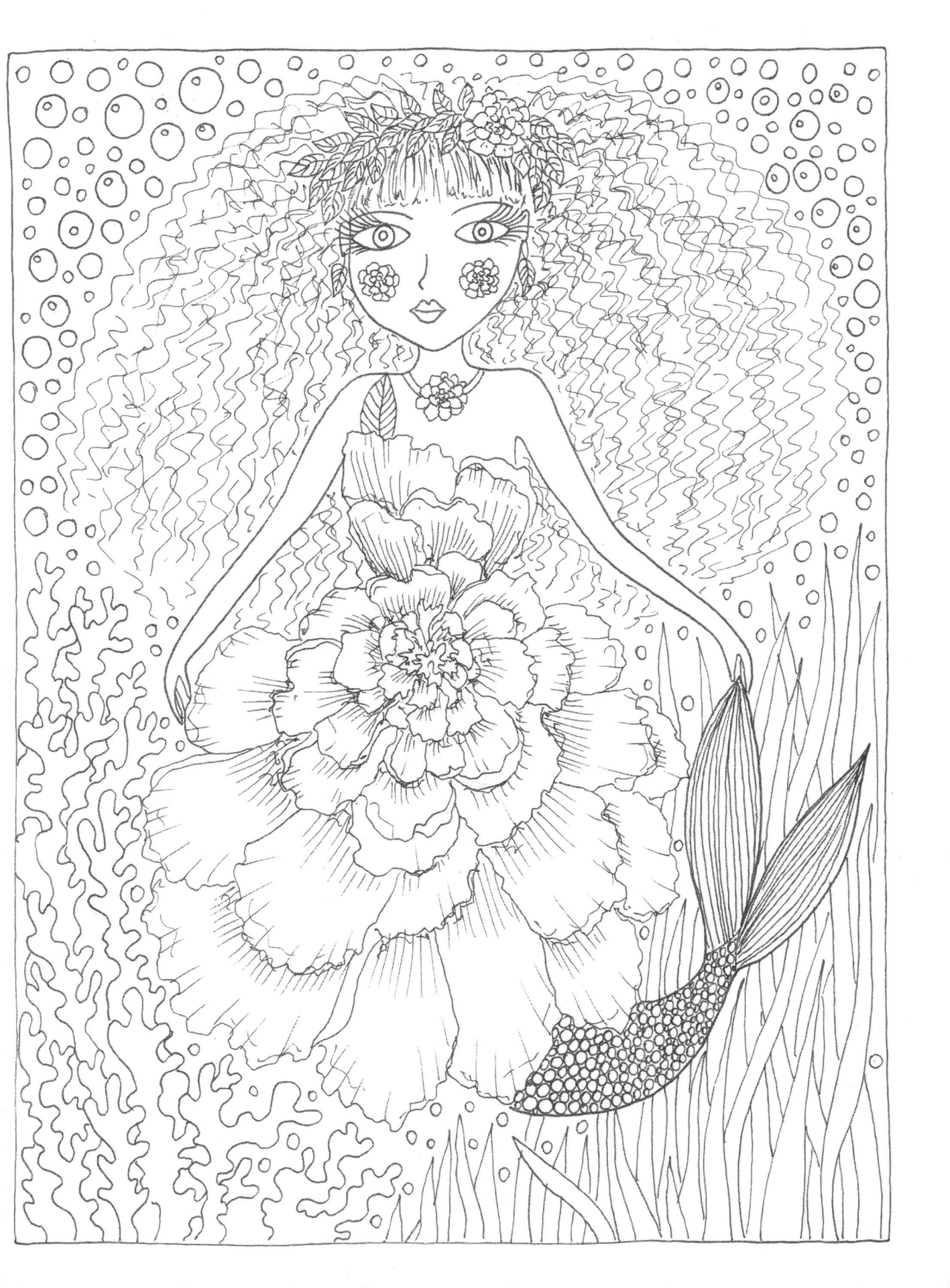

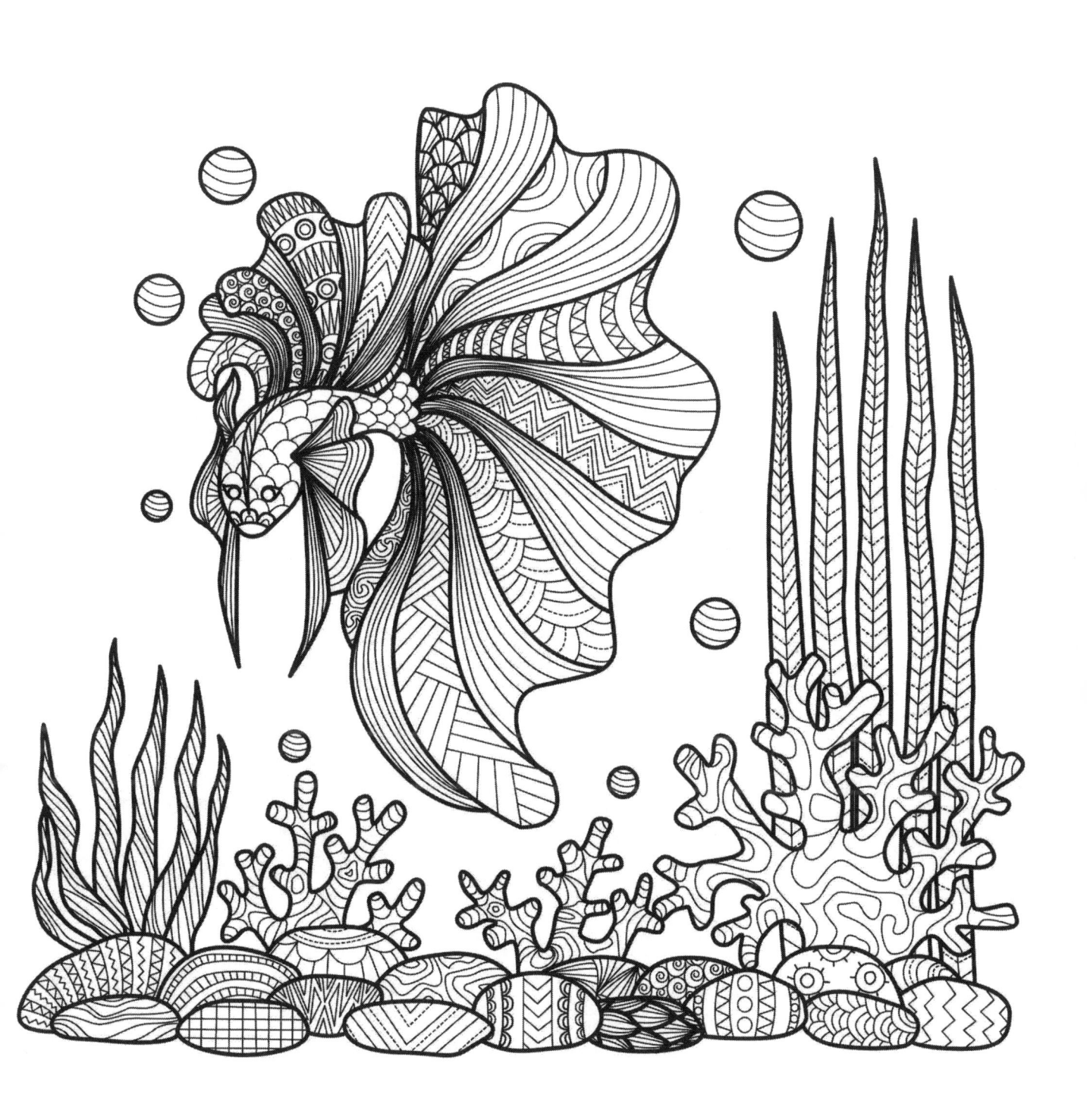

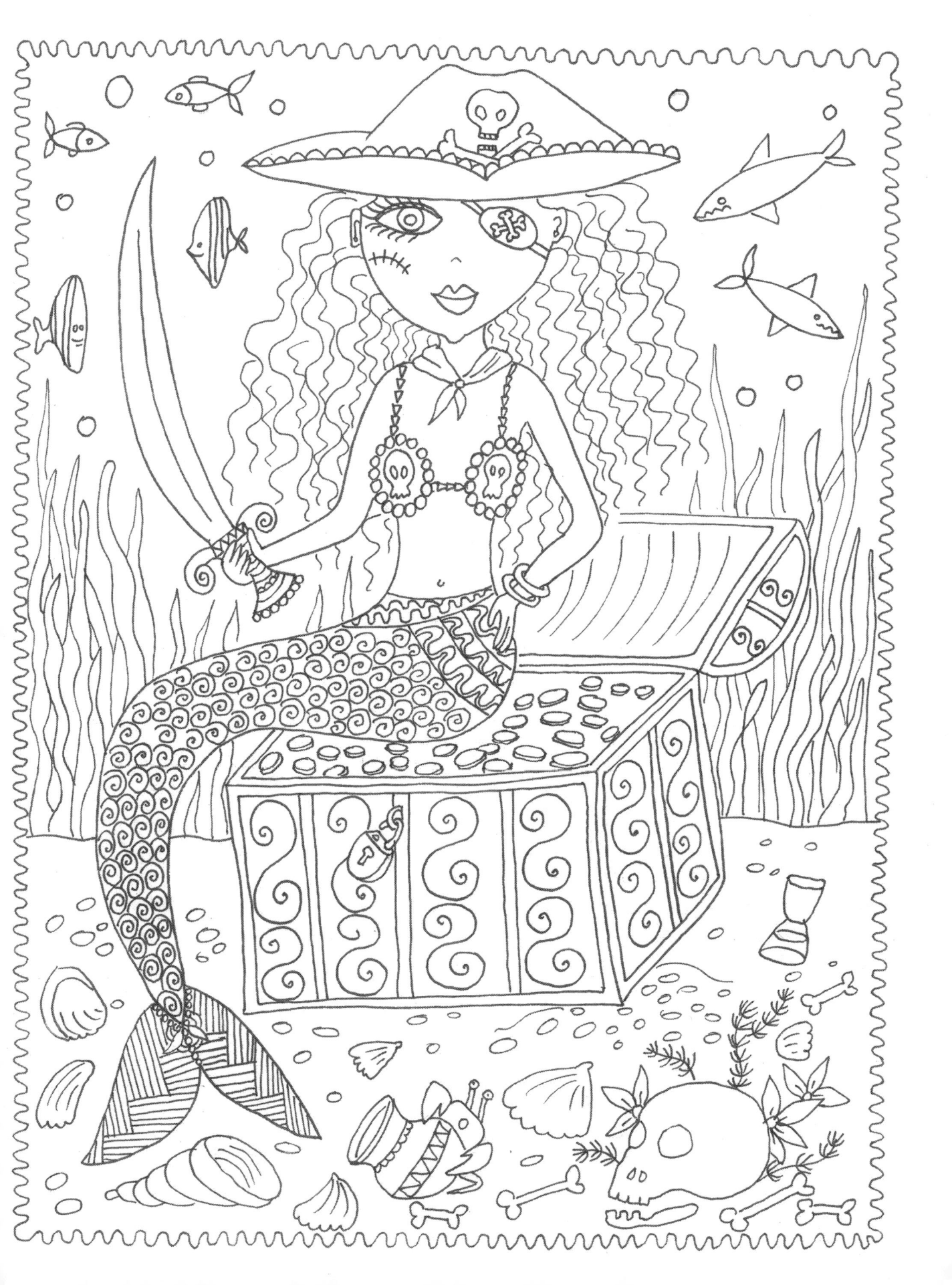

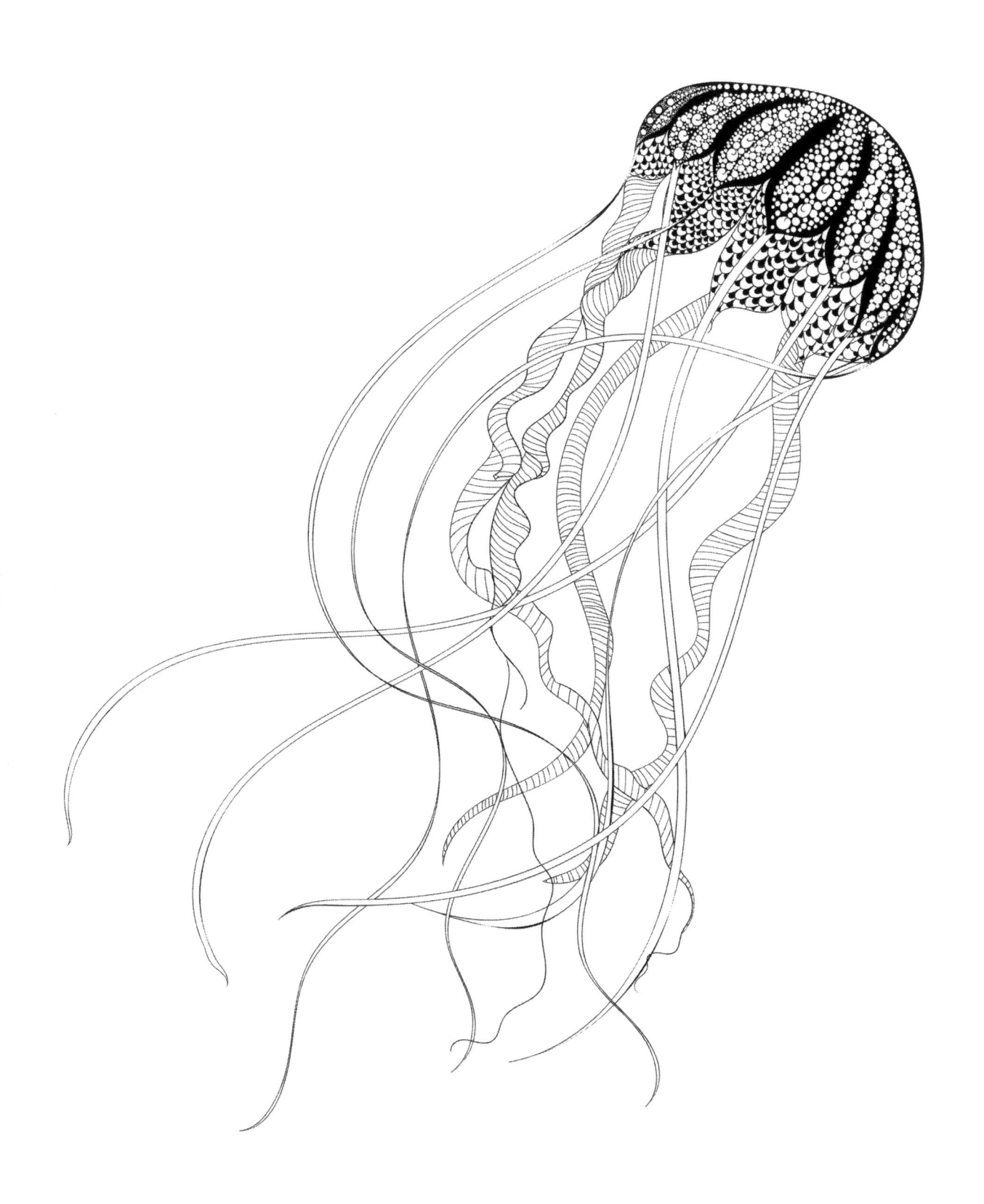

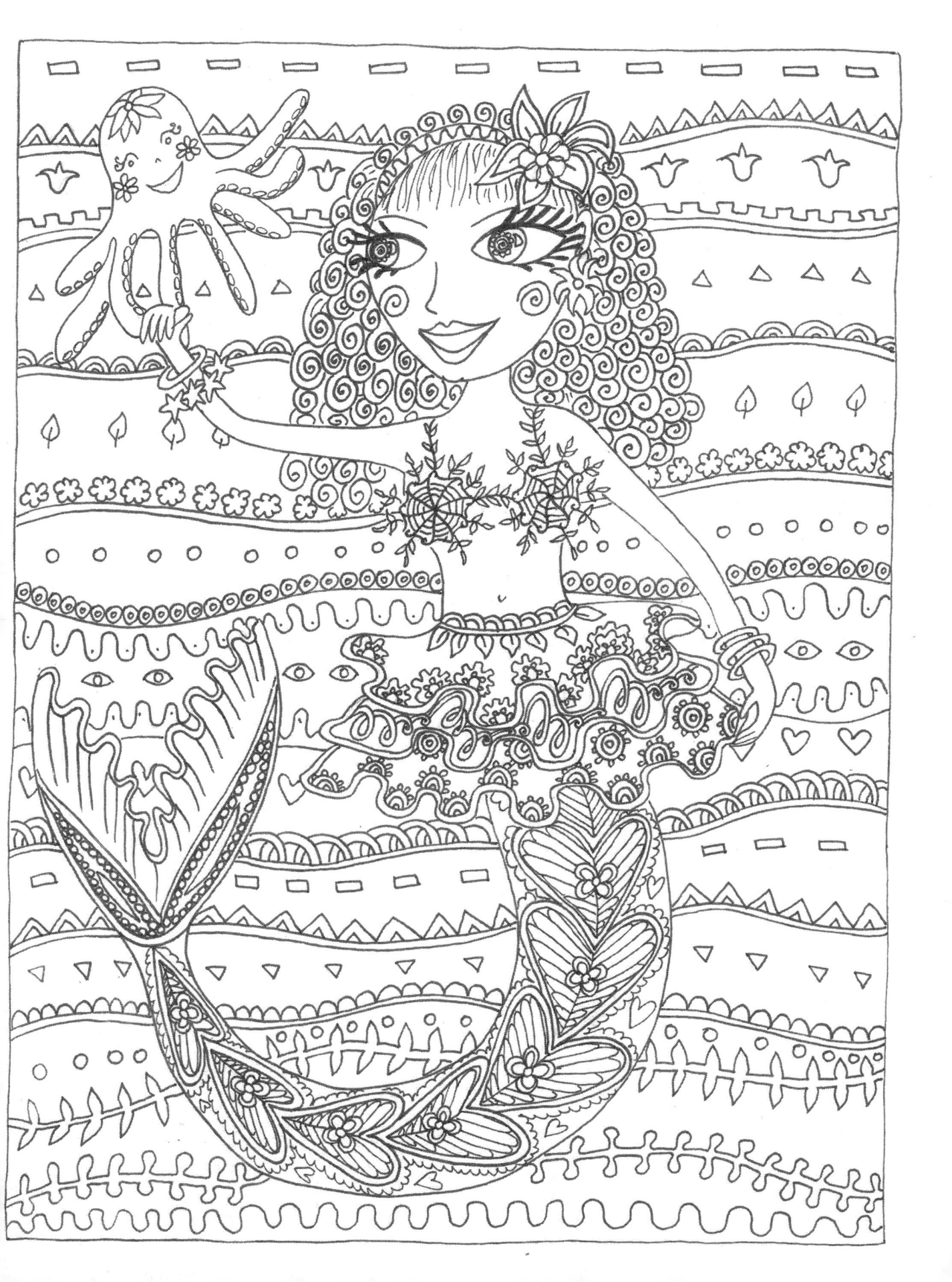

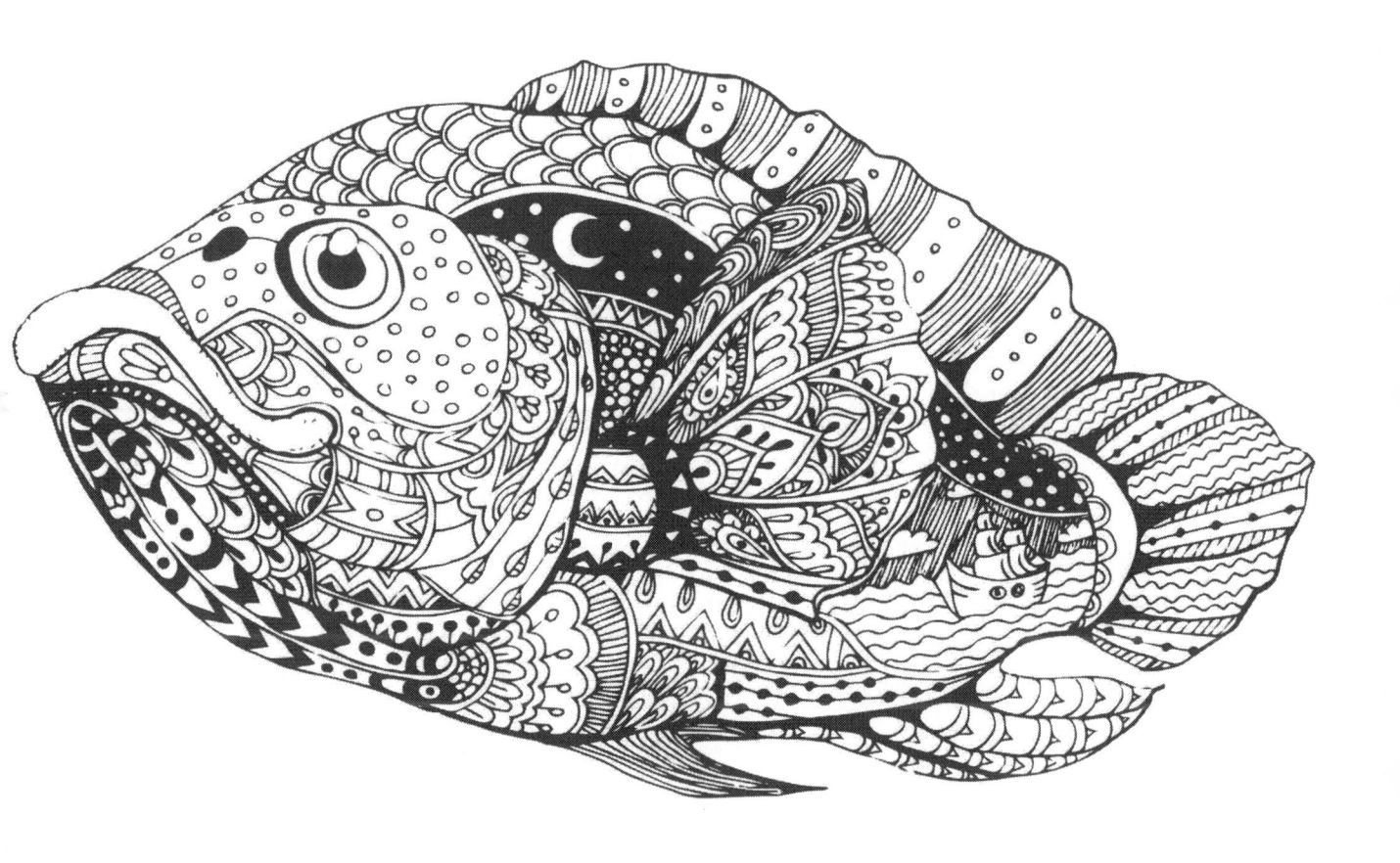

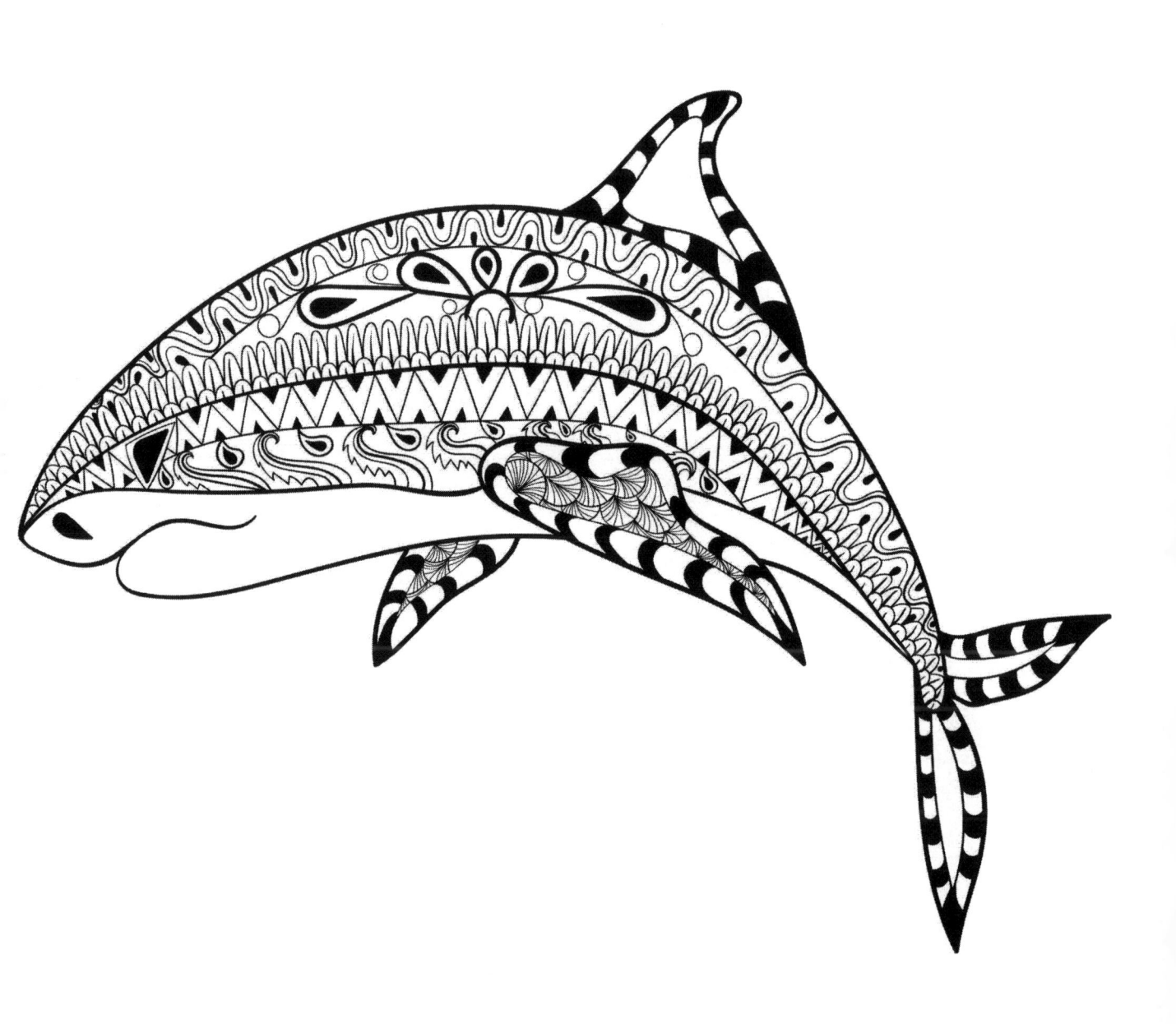

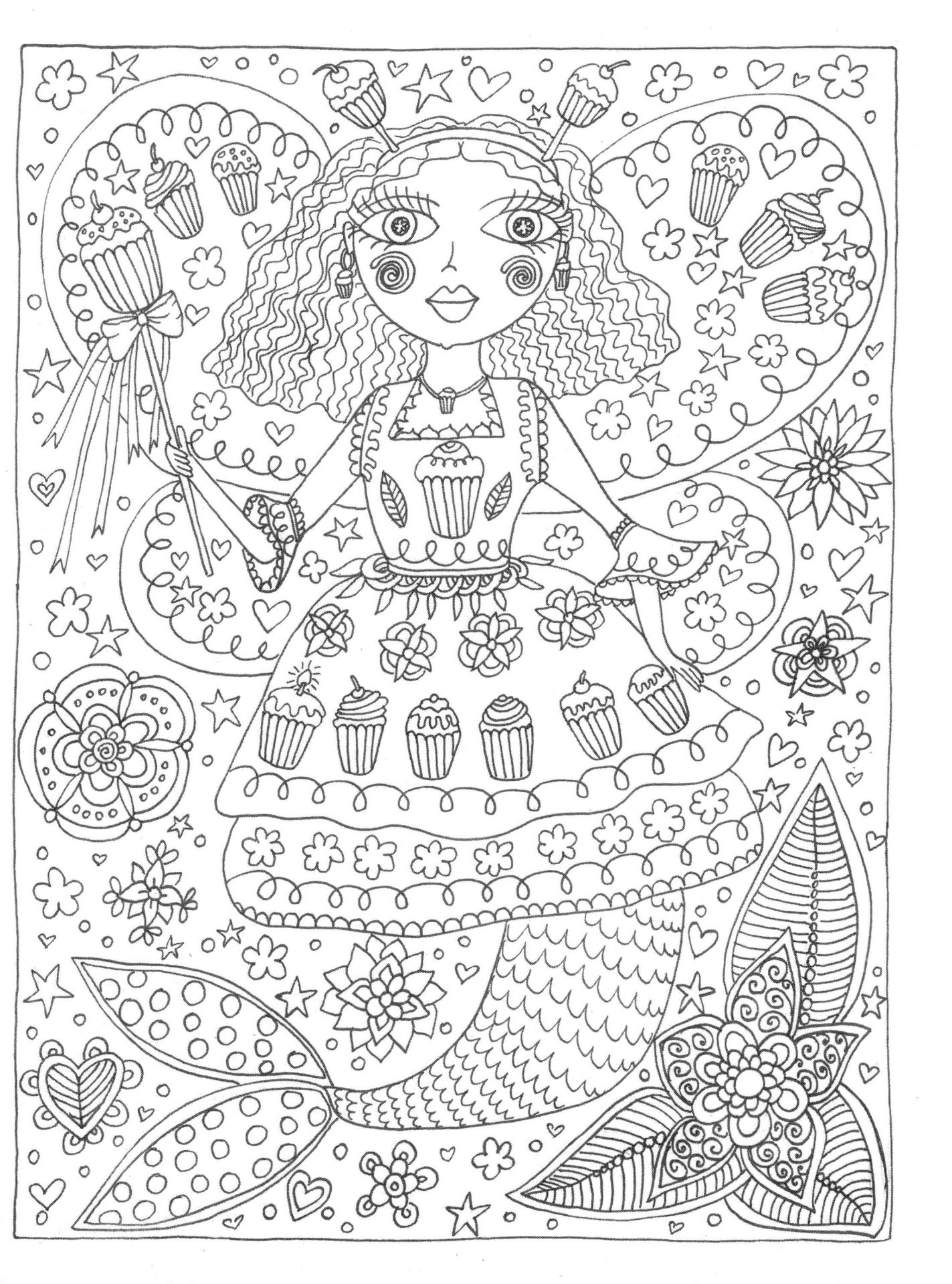

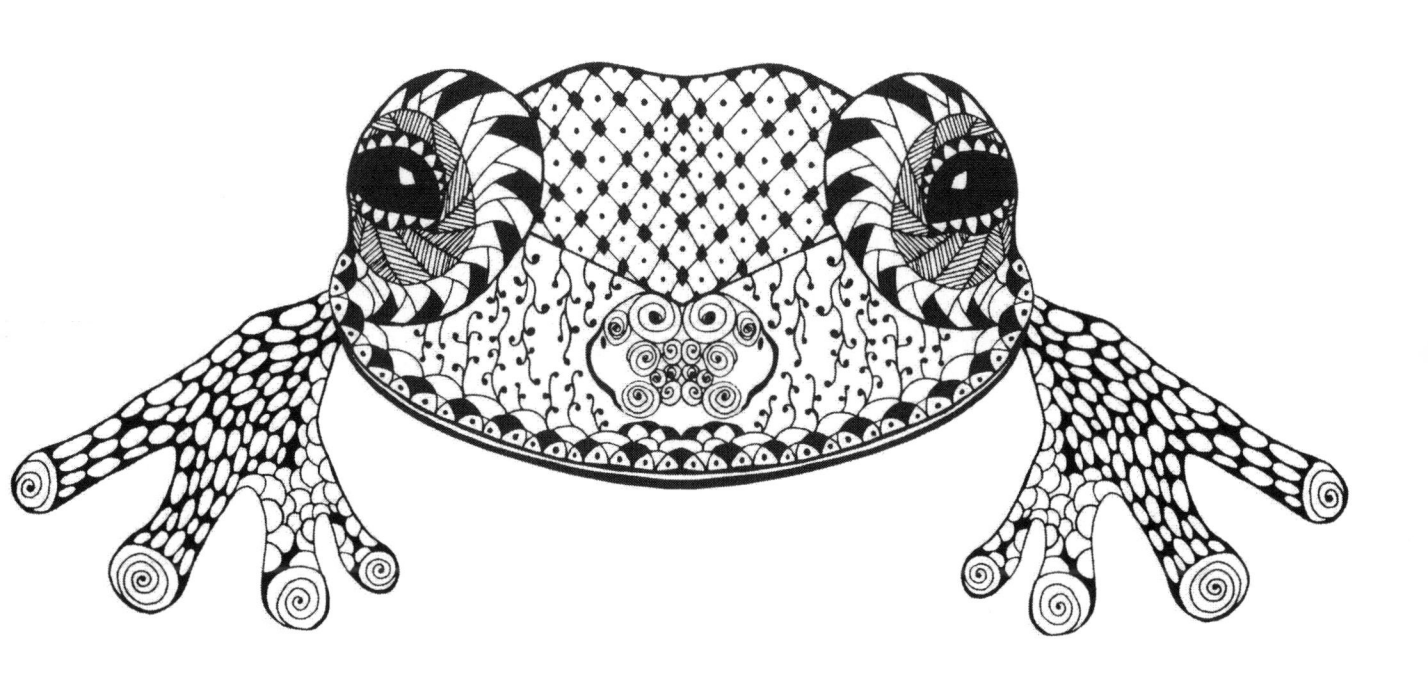

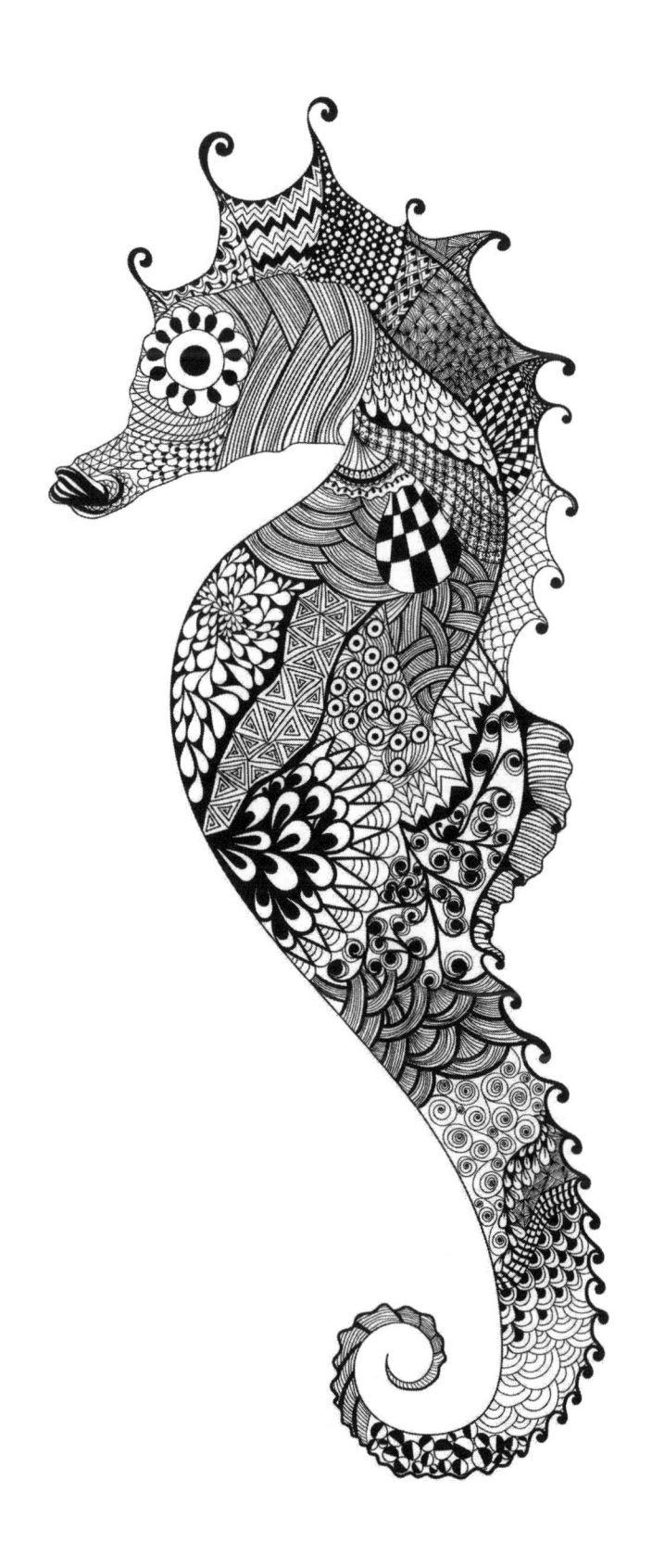

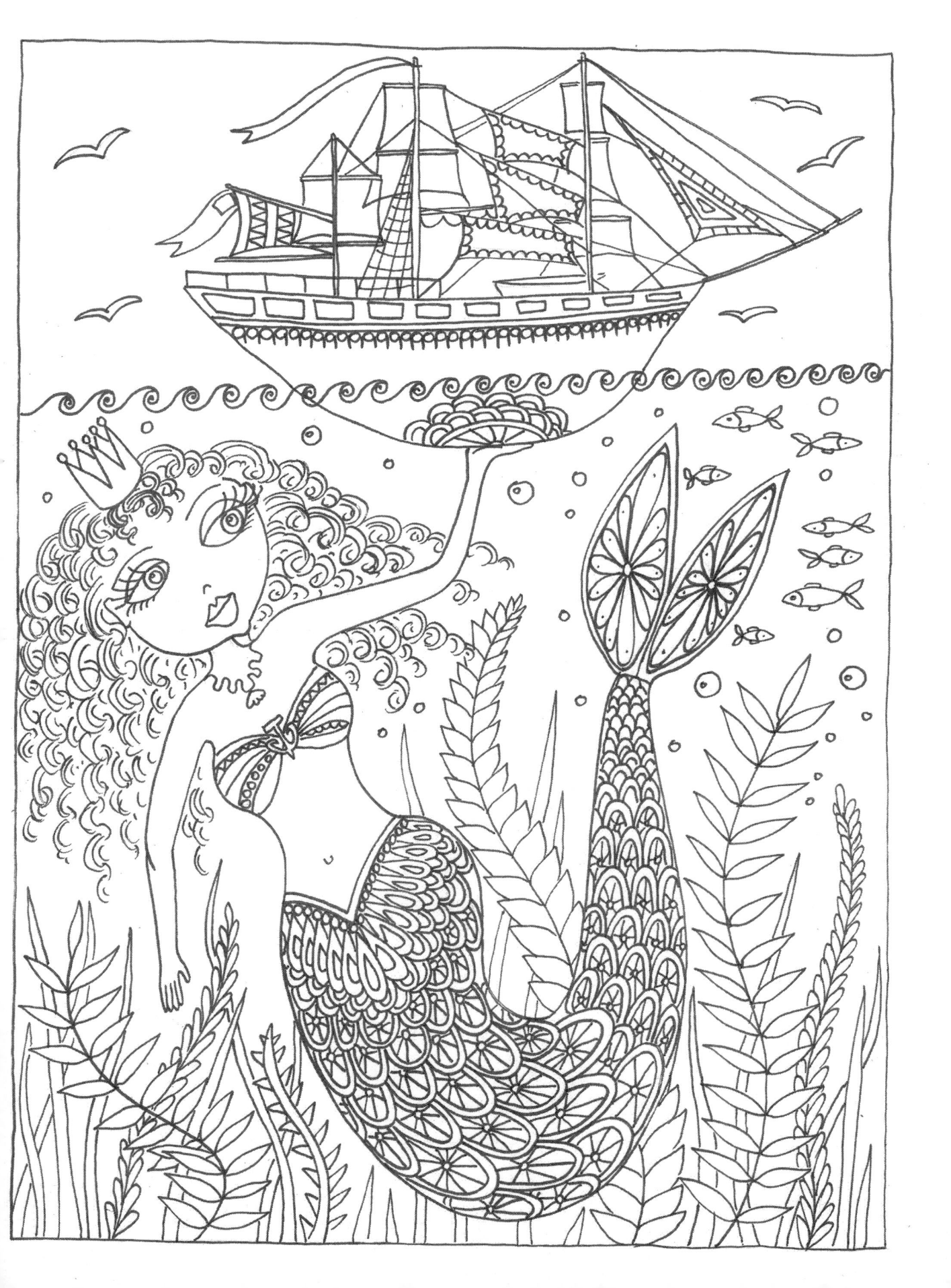

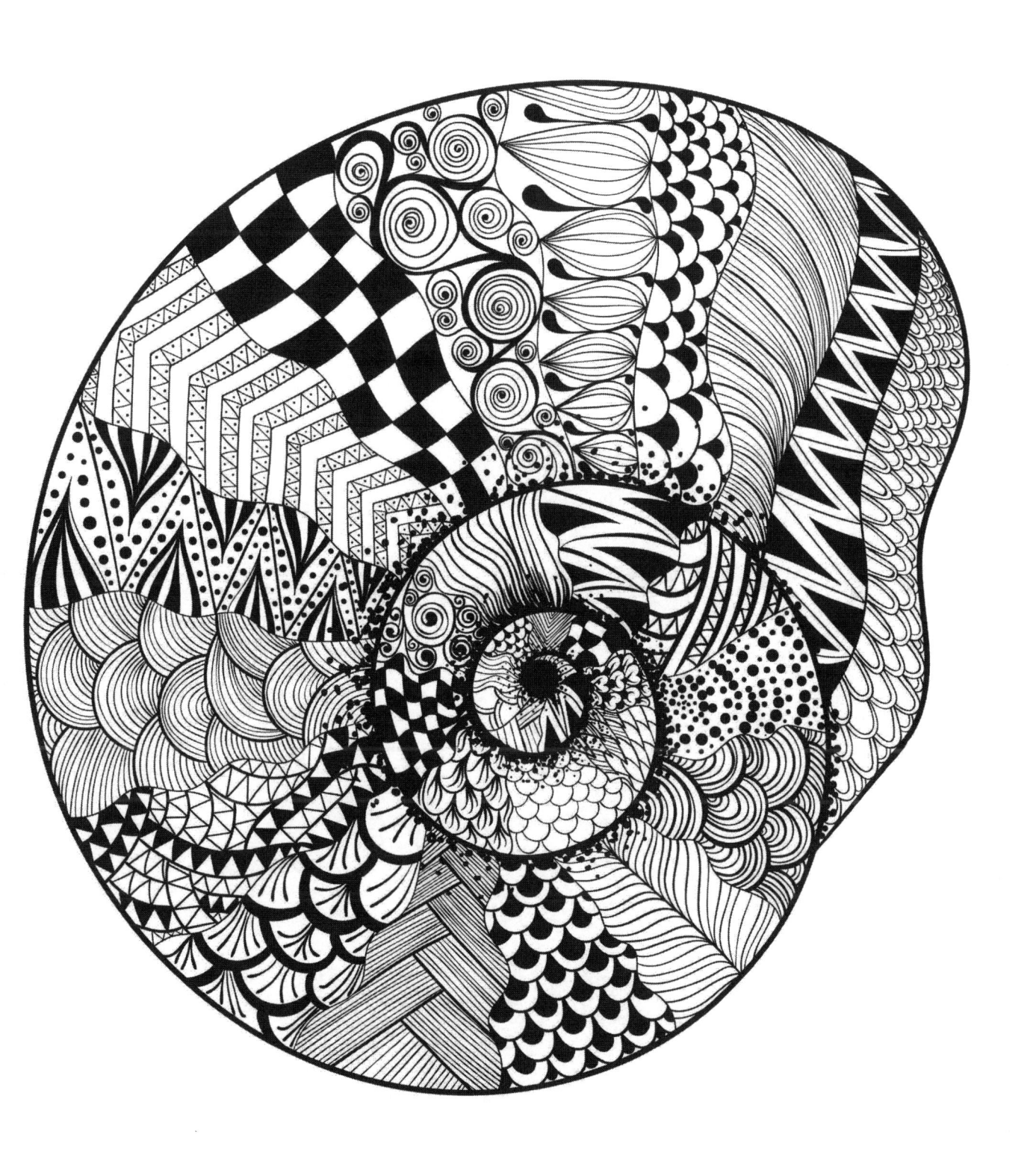

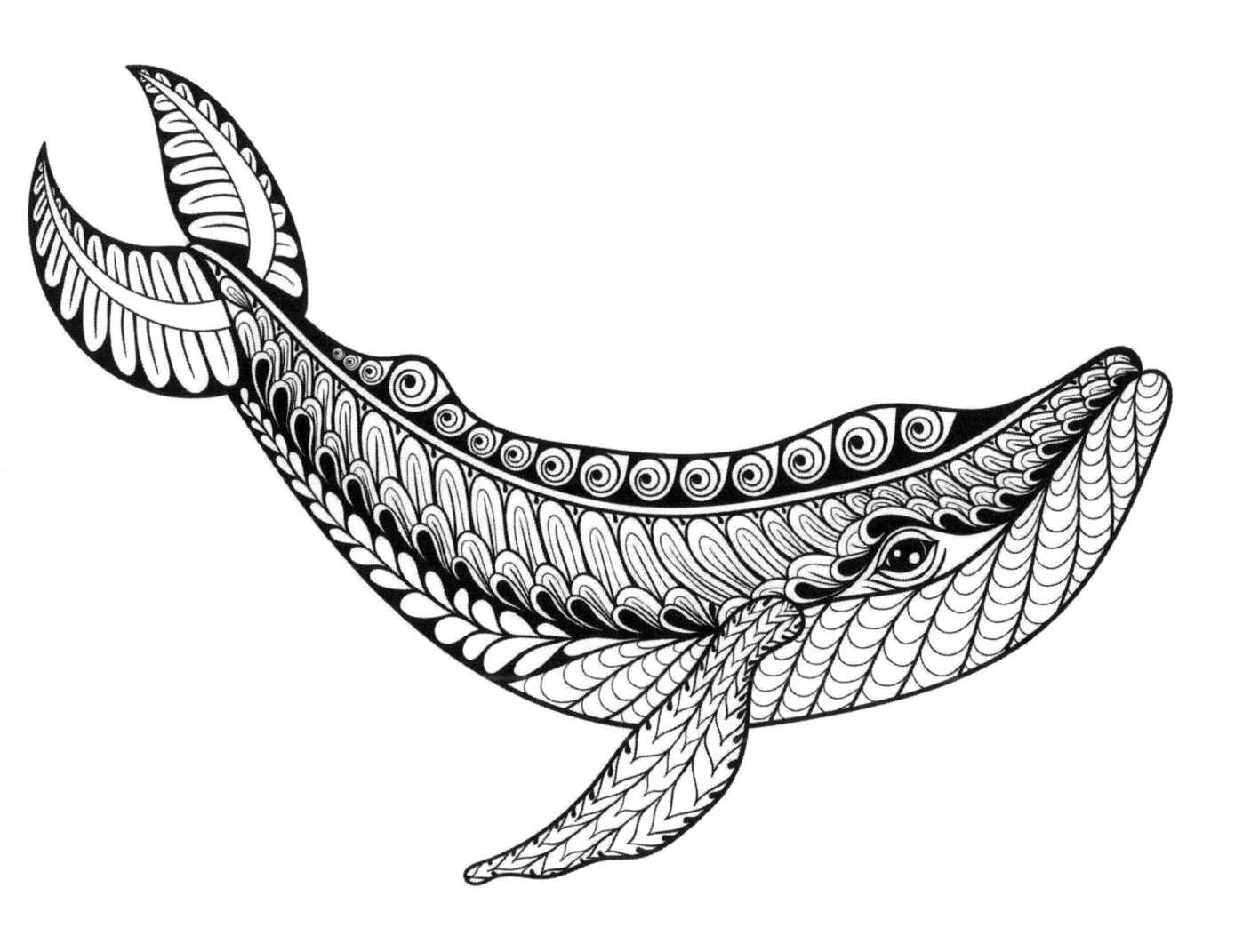

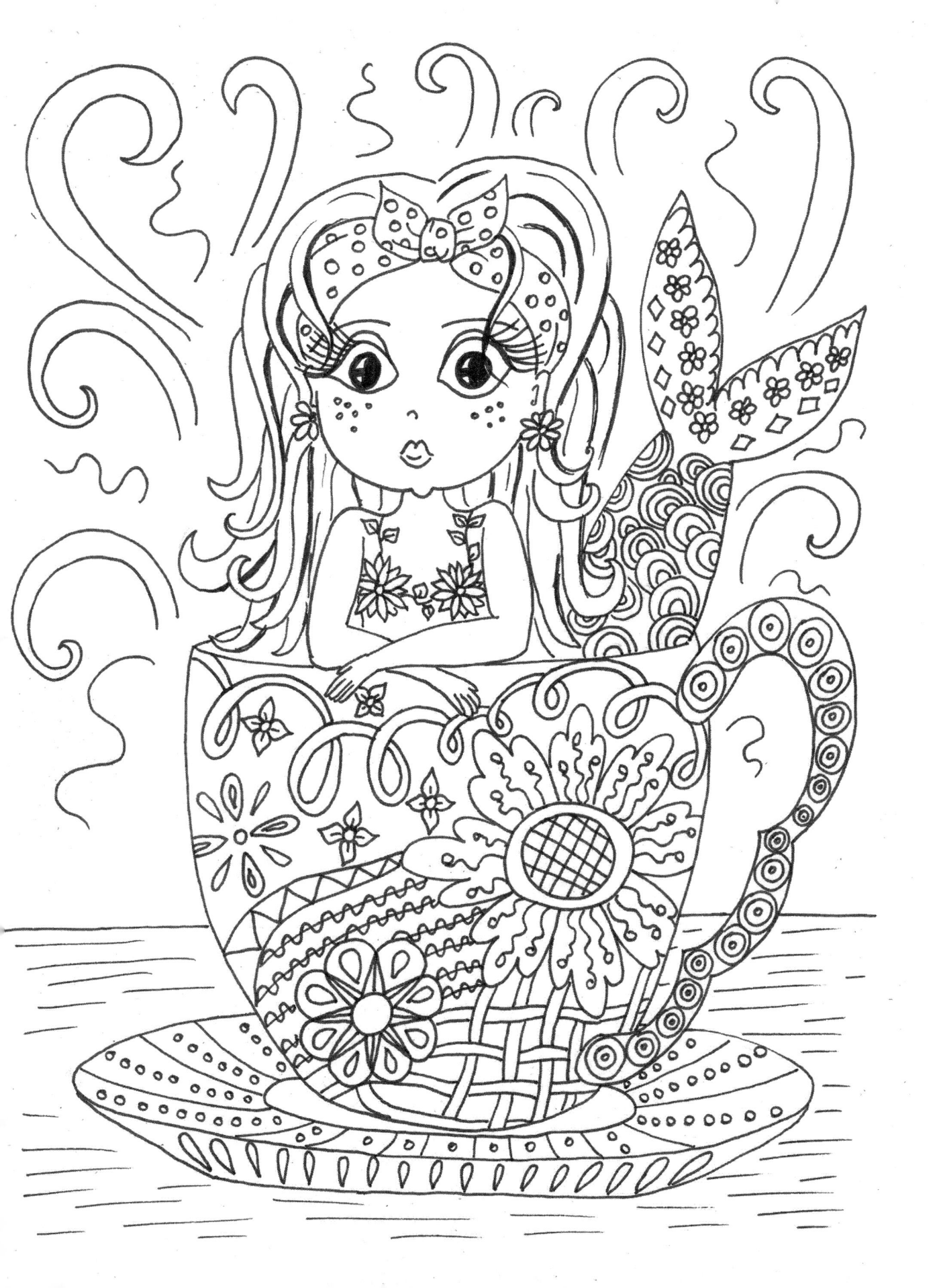

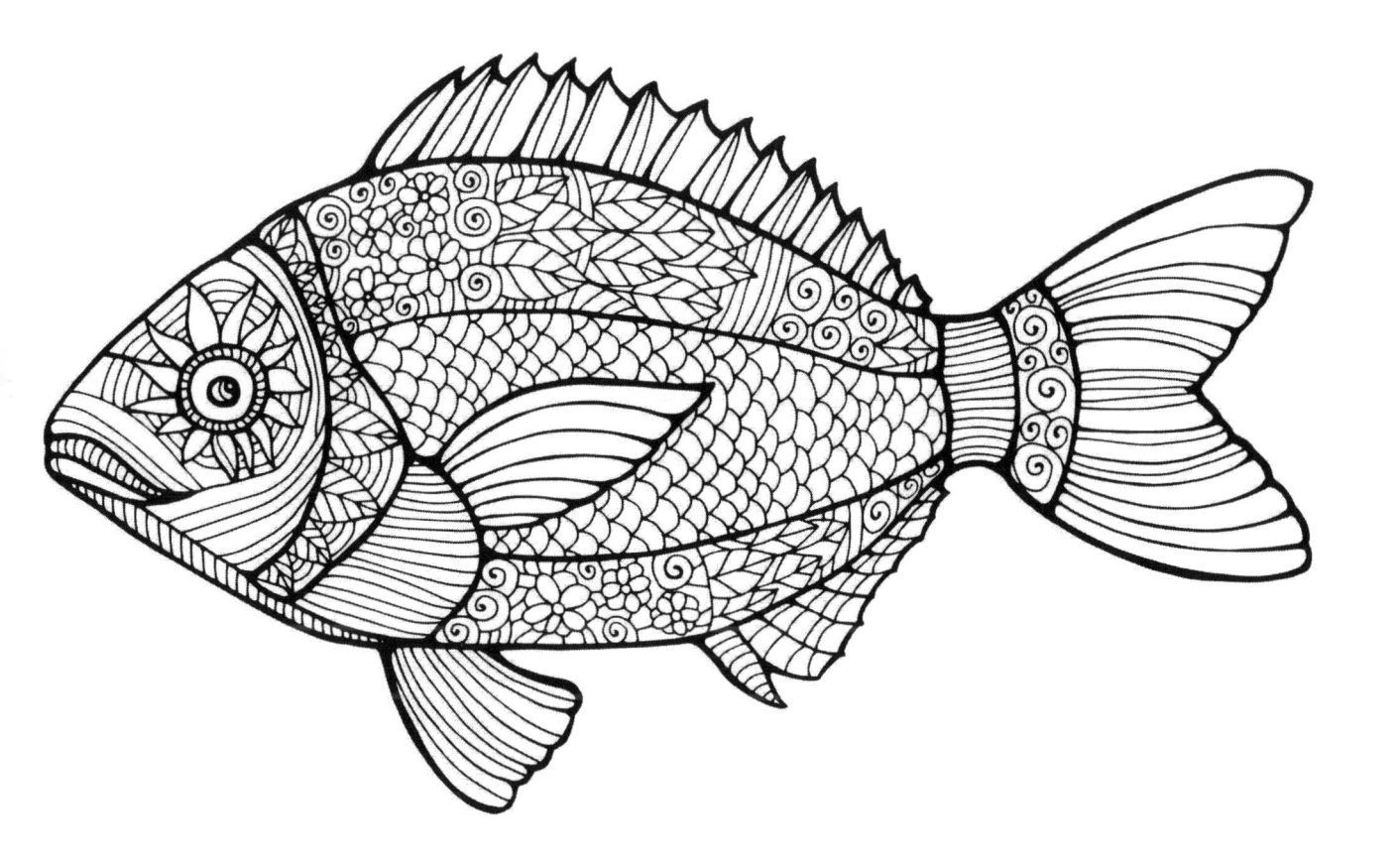

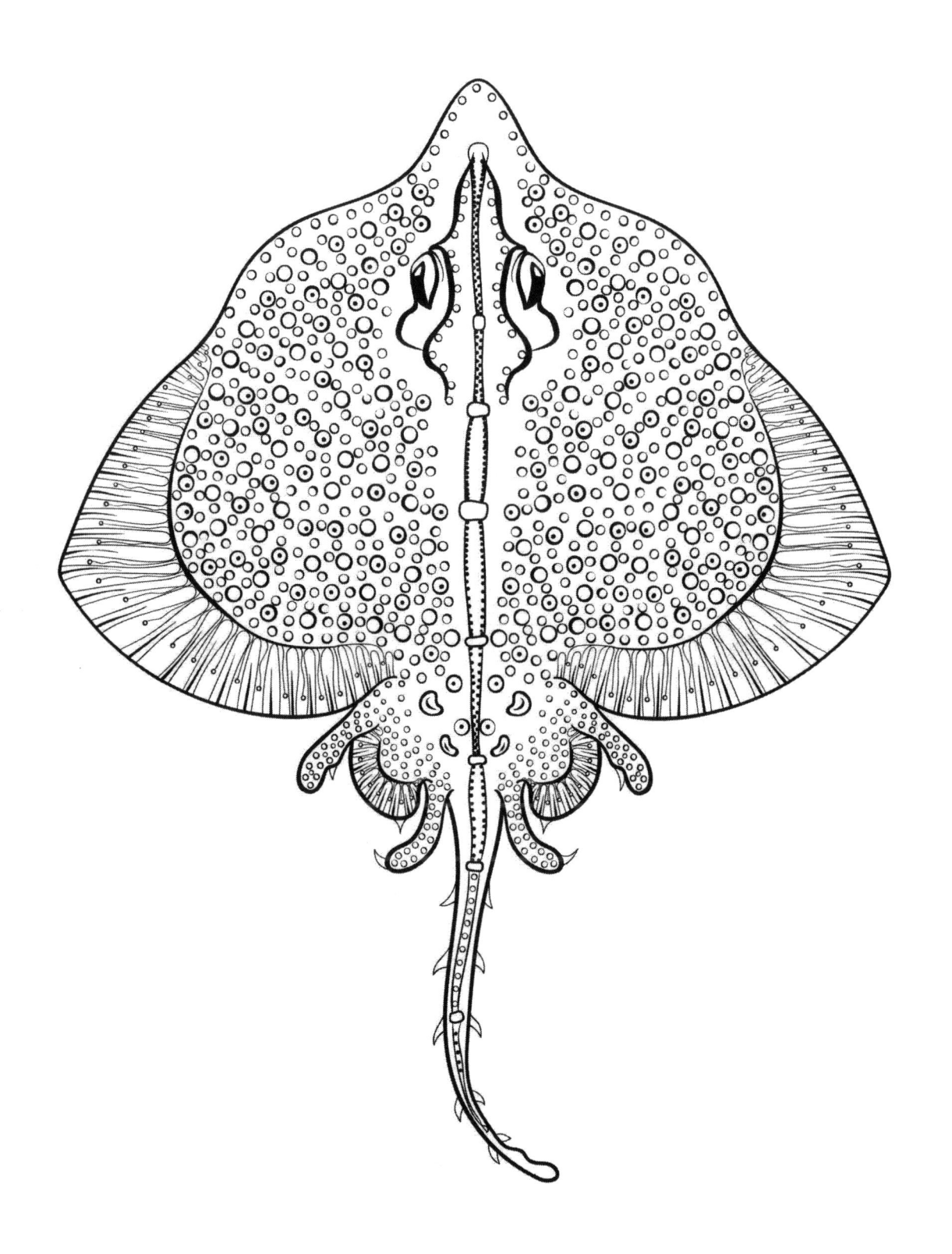

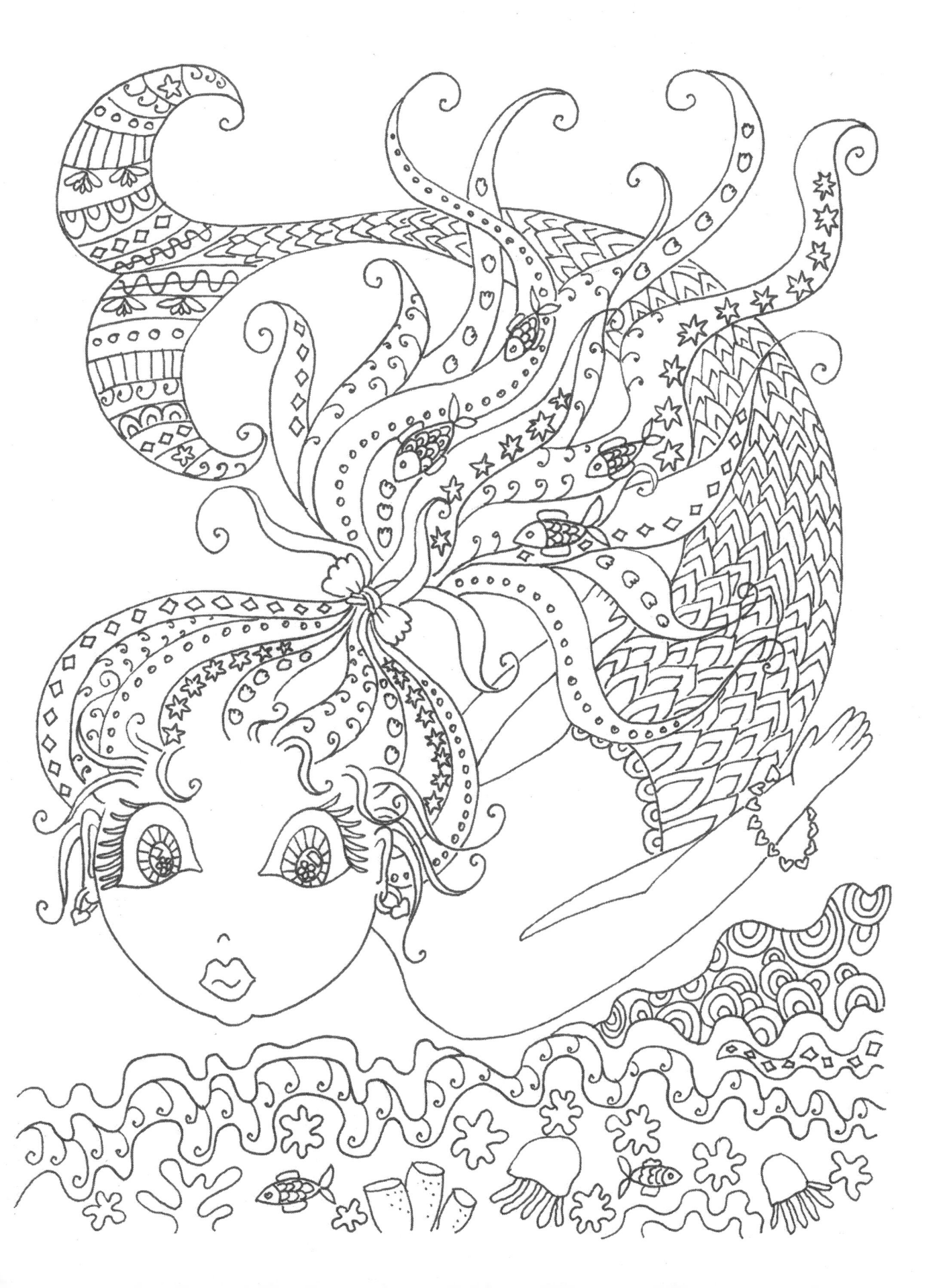

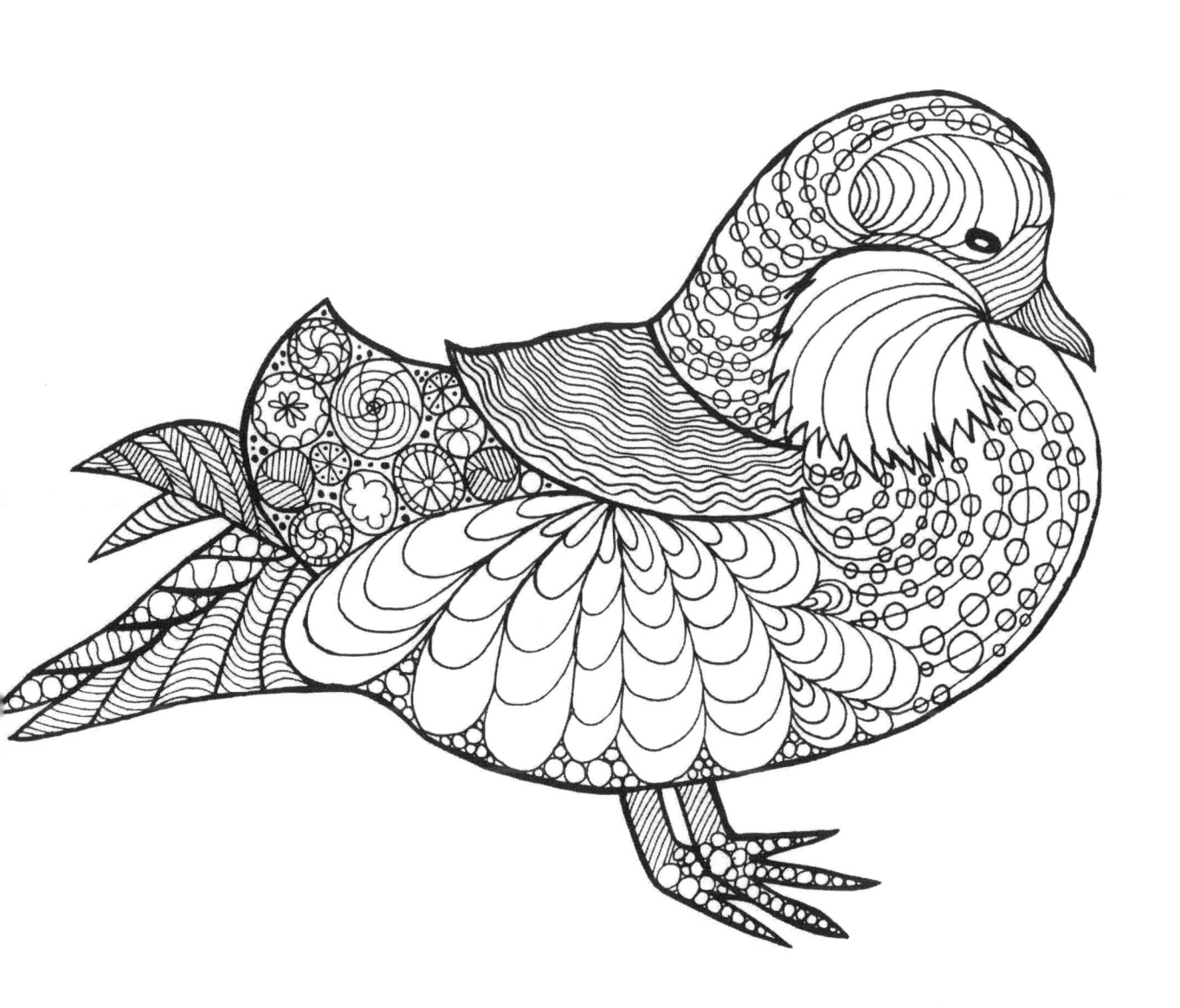

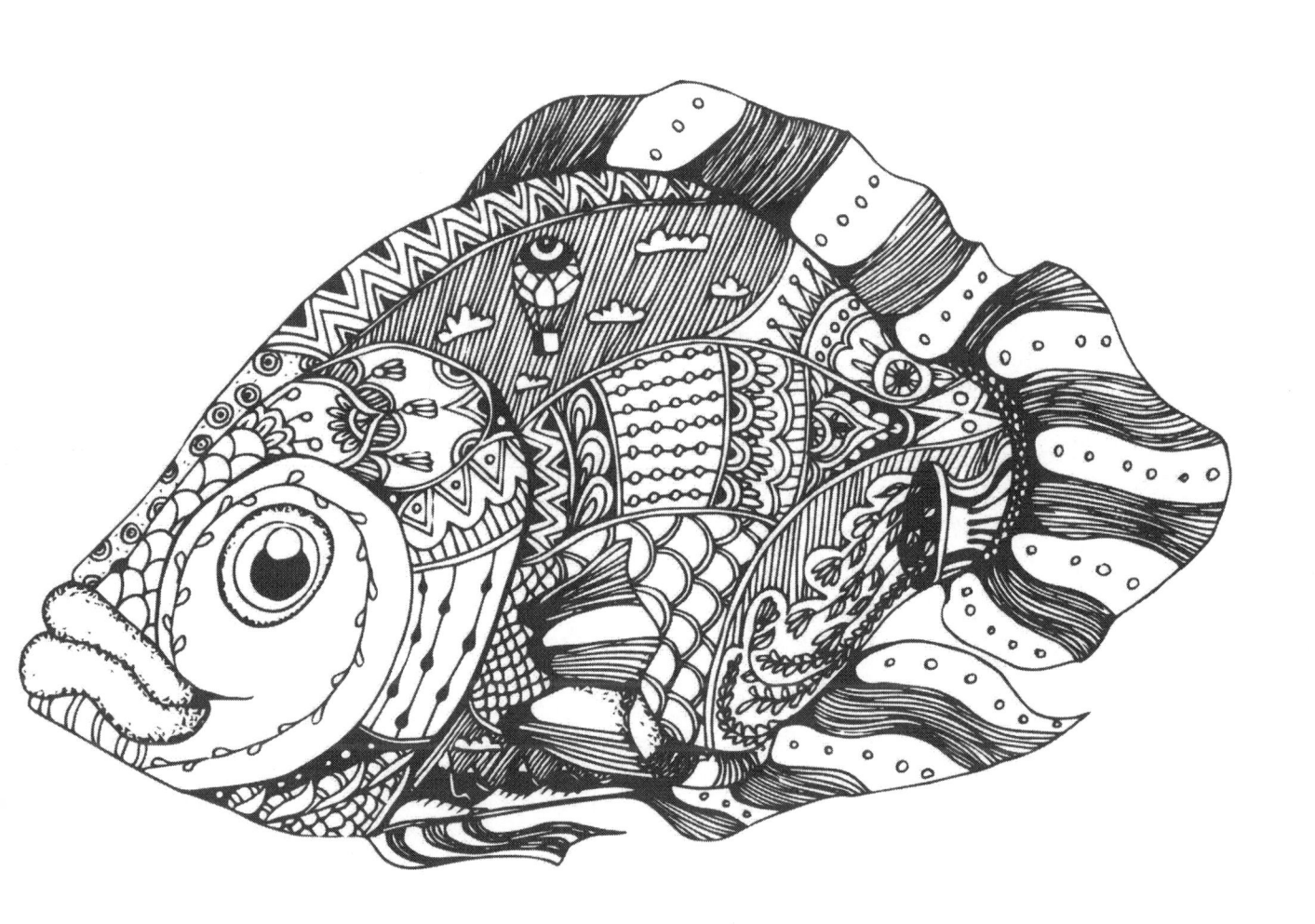

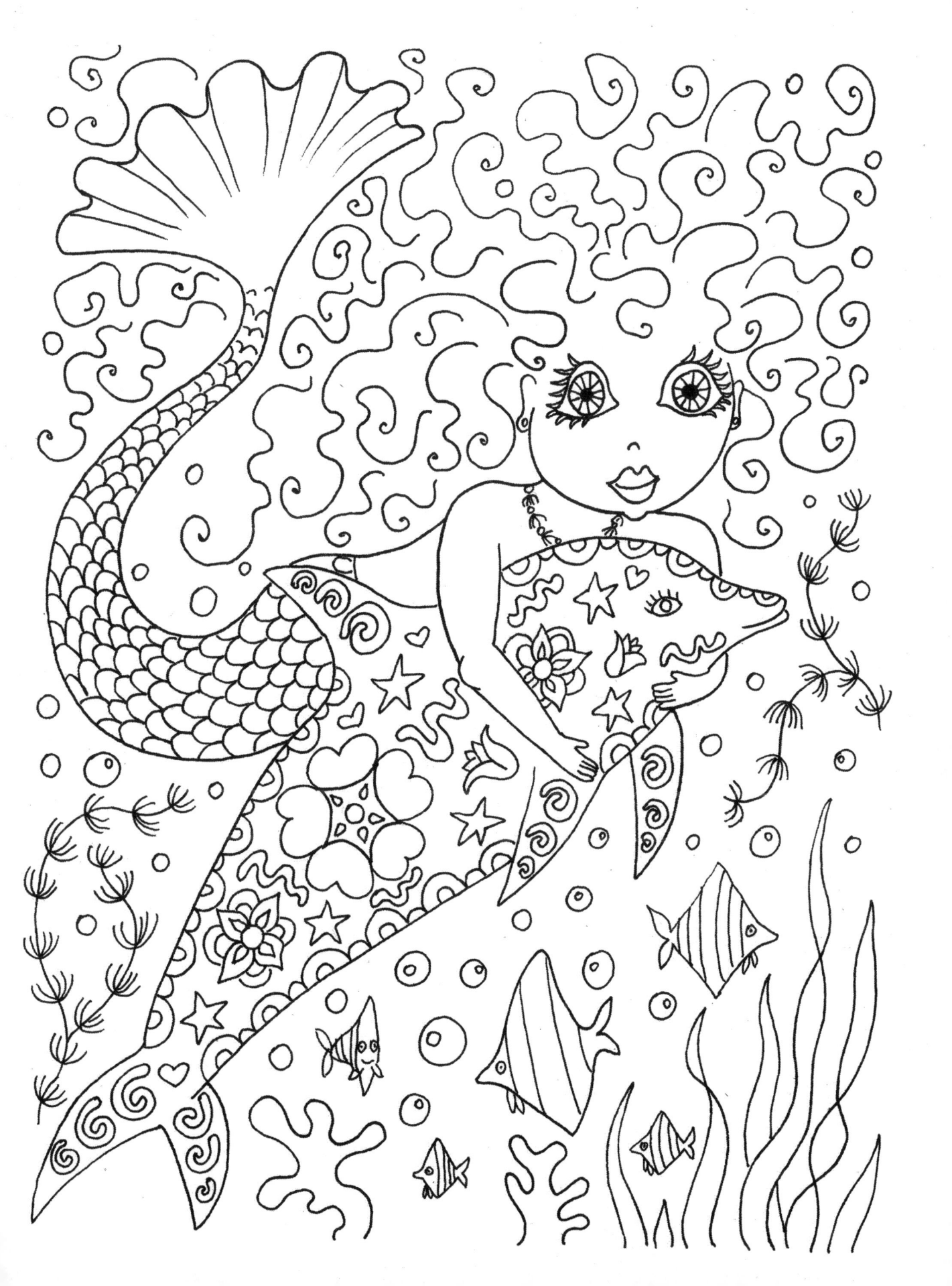

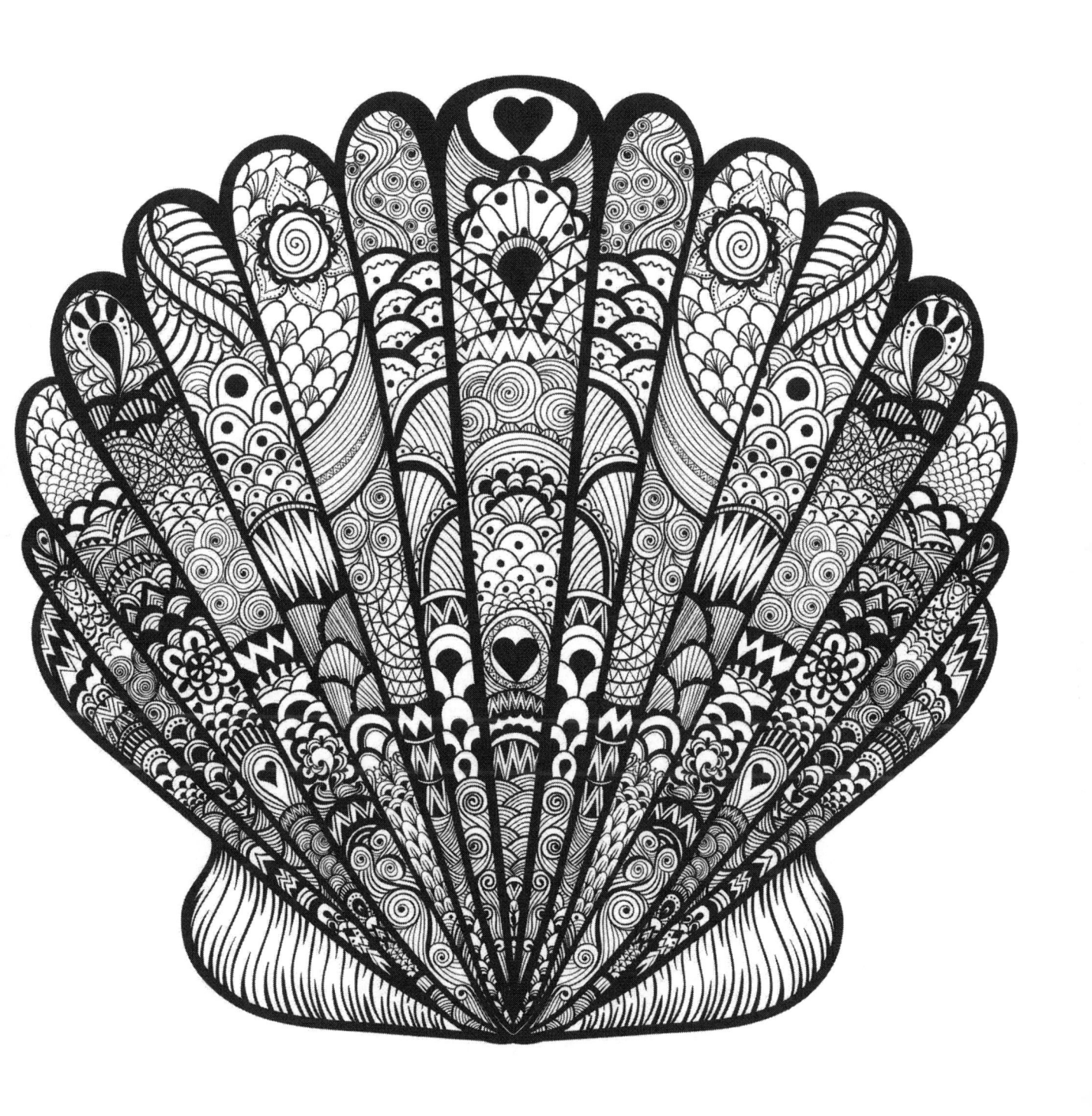

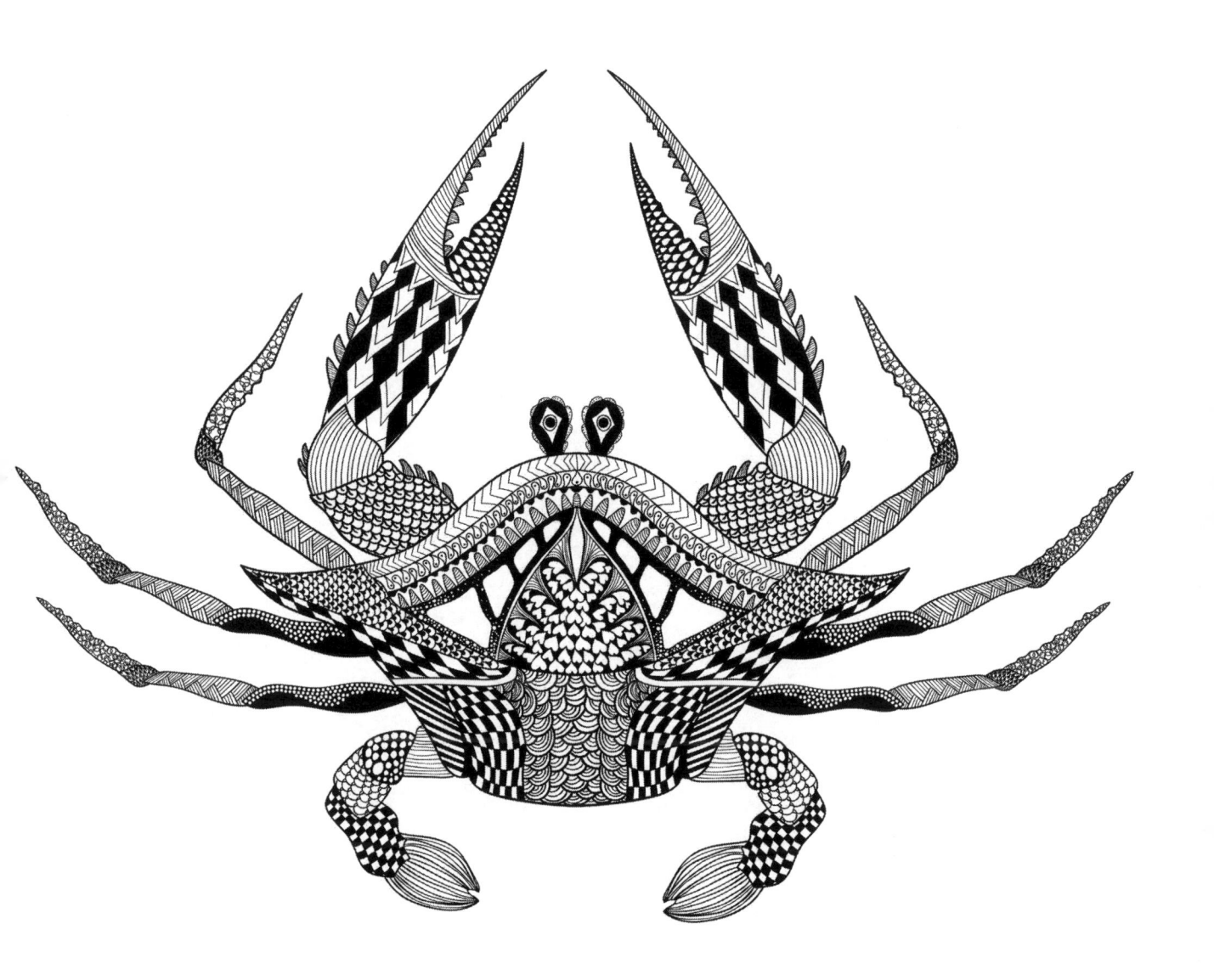

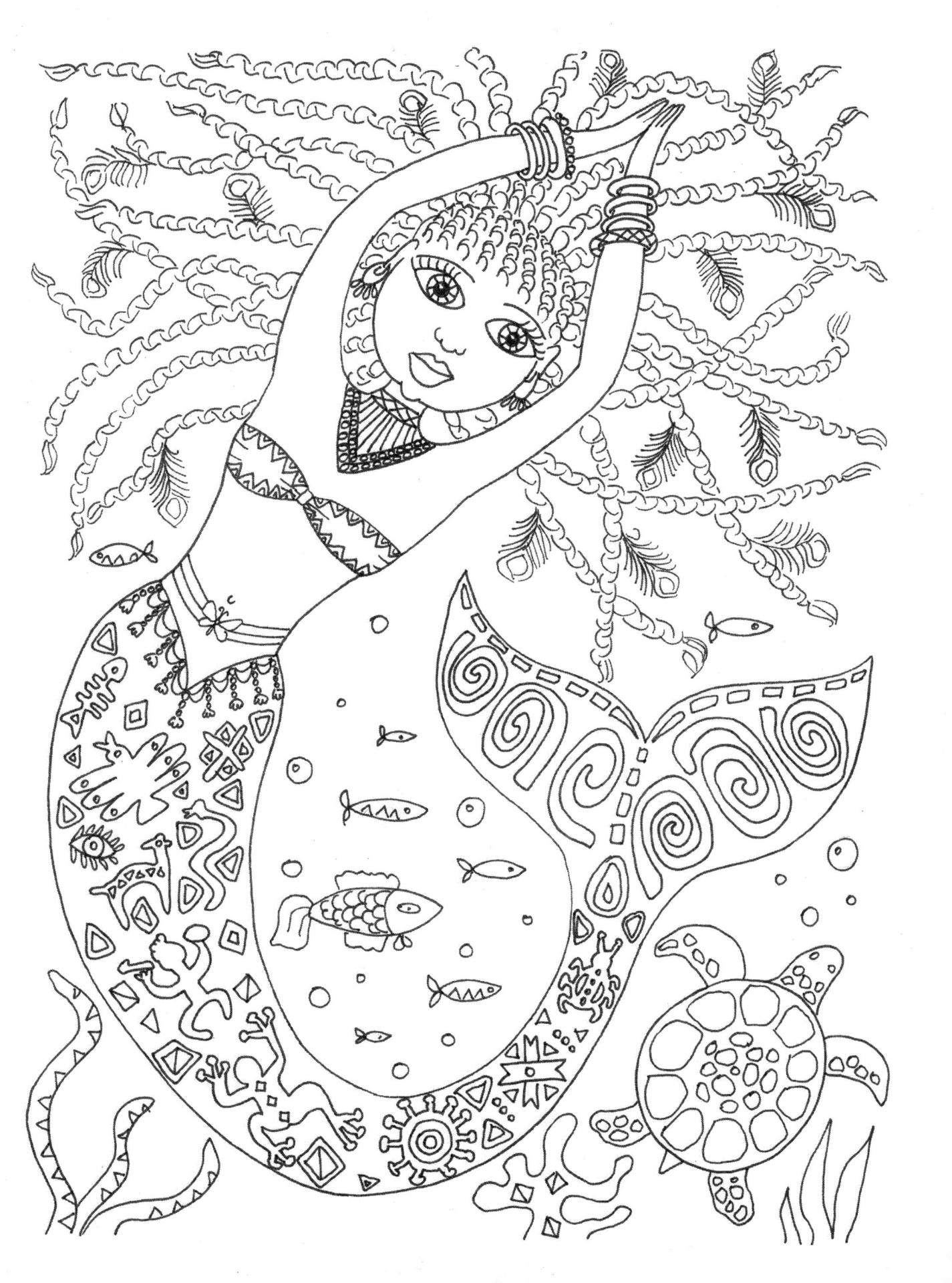

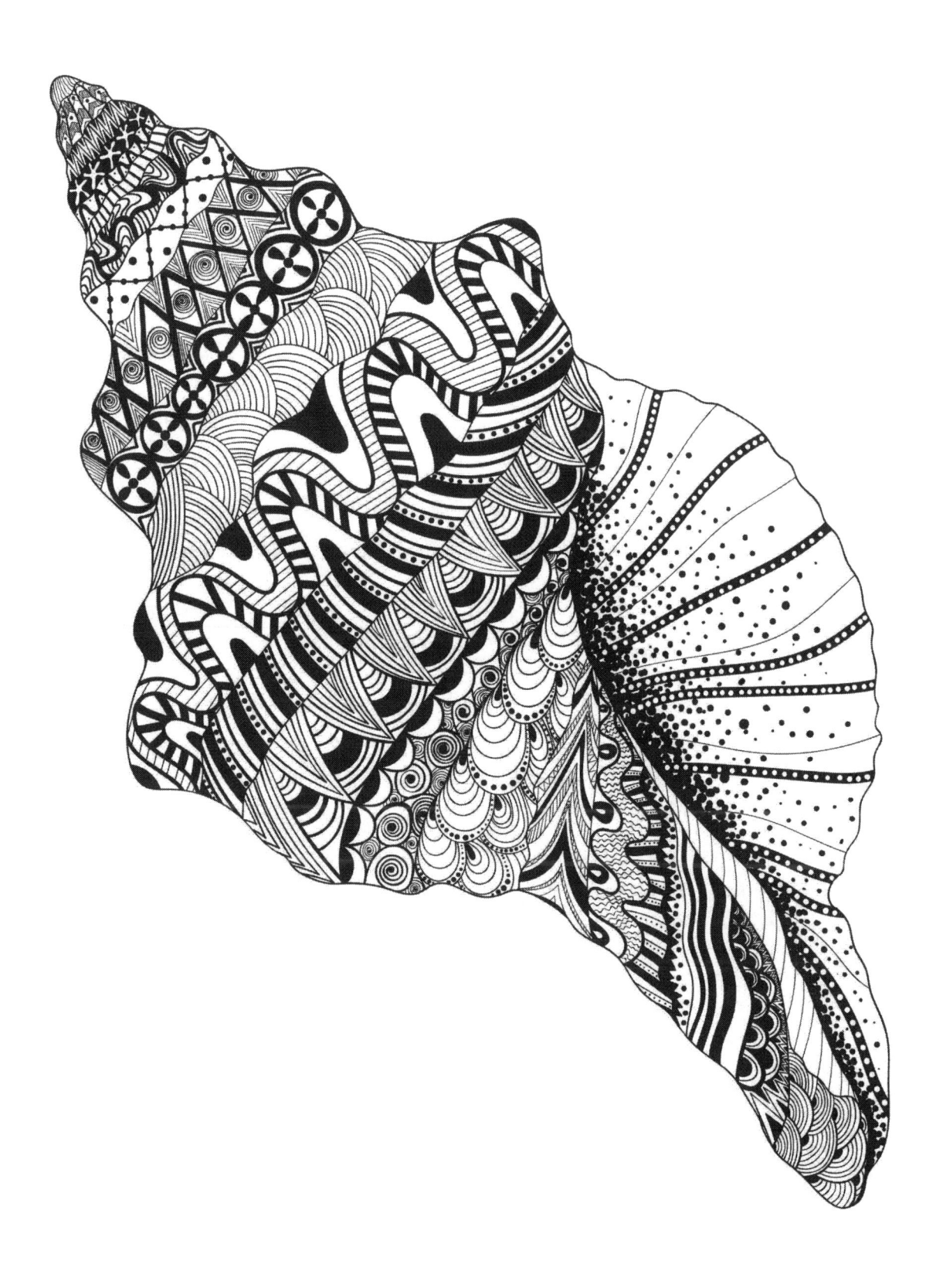

43846926R00047

Made in the USA
Middletown, DE
20 May 2017

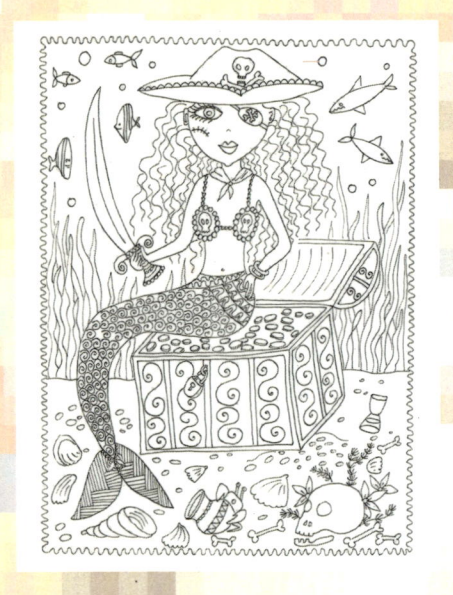
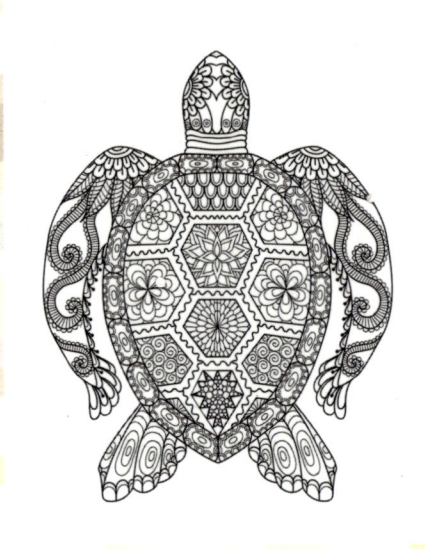
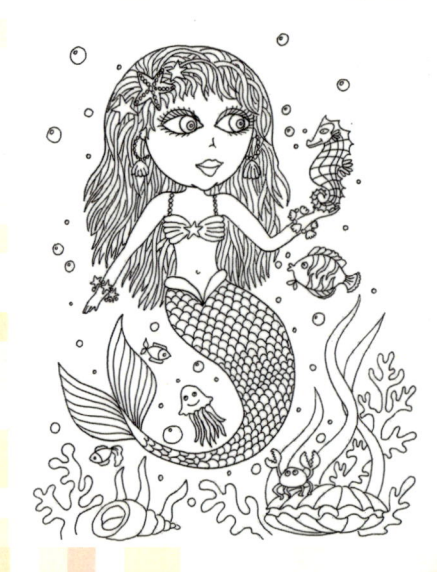

A Nice assortment of 40 mermaid and marine animal illustrations

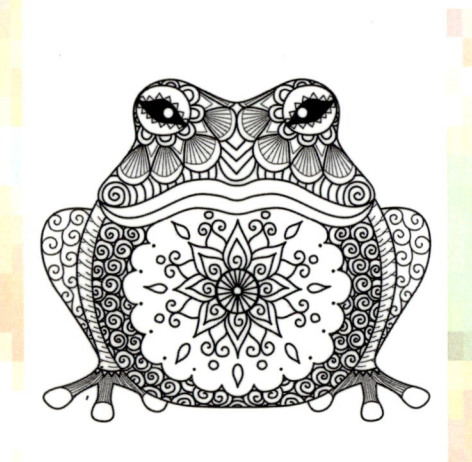
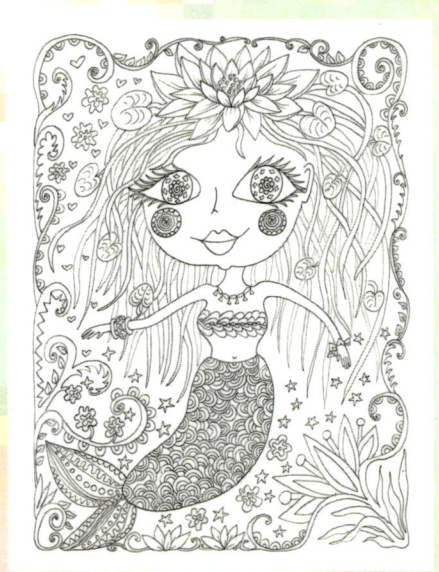
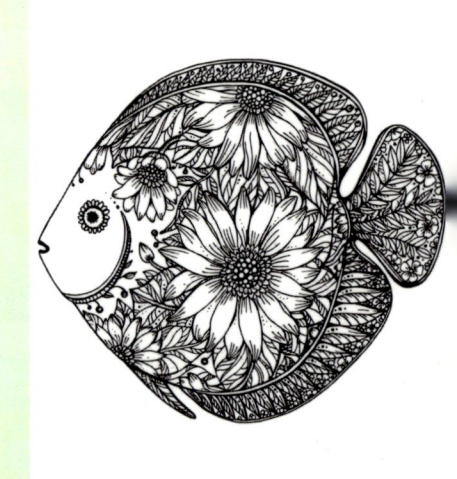

ISBN 9781988245225

90000

9 781988 245225